Infectious Disease: A Very Short Introduction

'This book provides a welcome introduction to infectious diseases that emphasizes an unusual perspective: the ecology and evolution of the pathogens responsible. This will be enlightening to newcomers to the topic as well as to those whose perspective on infections focuses on the public health and medical aspects.'

Marc Lipsitch, Professor of Epidemiology,
Harvard T. H. Chan School of Public Health

'An up-to-date summary of the relevant concepts applied to the specific details of important infectious diseases.'

Dieter Ebert, Professor of Zoology
and Evolutionary Biology, Universität Basel

VERY SHORT INTRODUCTIONS are for anyone wanting a stimulating and accessible way into a new subject. They are written by experts, and have been translated into more than 40 different languages.

The series began in 1995, and now covers a wide variety of topics in every discipline. The VSI library now contains over 350 volumes—a Very Short Introduction to everything from Psychology and Philosophy of Science to American History and Relativity—and continues to grow in every subject area.

Very Short Introductions available now:

For more information visit our website

www.oup.com/vsi/

Marta L. Wayne and Benjamin M. Bolker

INFECTIOUS DISEASE

A Very Short Introduction

OXFORD
UNIVERSITY PRESS

Great Clarendon Street, Oxford, OX2 6DP,
United Kingdom

Oxford University Press is a department of the University of Oxford.
It furthers the University's objective of excellence in research, scholarship,
and education by publishing worldwide. Oxford is a registered trade mark of
Oxford University Press in the UK and in certain other countries

First edition published in 2015

Impression: 1

Published in the United States of America by Oxford University Press
198 Madison Avenue, New York, NY 10016, United States of America

British Library Cataloguing in Publication Data

Data available

Library of Congress Control Number: 2014959023

ISBN 978-0-19-968893-7

Printed in Great Britain by
Ashford Colour Press Ltd, Gosport, Hampshire

Contents

Acknowledgements

For Charlie, Norma, Tara, and (*in memoriam*) Django.

We acknowledge the partial support of the US National Institutes of Health. We would like to thank the understanding and professional editorial staff at Oxford University Press, especially Cathy Kennedy, along with our colleagues who contributed friendly reviews and technical advice: Rustom Antia, Janis Antonovics, Julia Buck, Robin Bush, Jonathan Dushoff, David Earn, David Hillis, Lindsay Keegan, Marm Kilpatrick, Aaron King, Marc Lipsitch, Glenn Morris, Juliet Pulliam, Marco Salemi, and David Smith. Needless to say, we are entirely responsible for any remaining errors or oversimplifications.

List of illustrations

Chapter 1
Introduction

We talk about 'infectious lyrics' and 'viral videos'. Metaphors of infectious disease saturate Western popular culture in the 21st century. Anxiety over the next pandemic simmers subliminally worldwide. Infectious disease crises come and go: over the past decade we have worried in turn about bioterrorism, SARS, H1N1 influenza, and the Ebola virus.

As recently as the 1970s, doctors were boldly proclaiming the beginning of the end for infectious disease. They thought their arsenal of vaccines for preventing viral diseases and broad-spectrum antibiotics for treating bacterial infections could handle any threat. But disease was never dead, or even in remission. Even as the doctors announced victory, drug resistant strains of *Staphylococcus aureus* (one of the 'flesh-eating bacteria' of British tabloids) were spreading in hospitals. (Japan had experienced outbreaks of drug resistant bacteria in the 1950s, but at the time these epidemics were little noticed in the West.) Things got worse as HIV, which has stubbornly resisted the development of vaccine to the present day, emerged in the 1980s. In recognition of the renewed threat of infectious disease, the US Institute of Medicine coined the phrase 'emerging and re-emerging diseases' in the early 1990s.

An infectious disease is one that you can catch from another person or organism as a result of the transmission of a biological agent. In contrast, you fall ill with non-infectious diseases—heart disease, diabetes, Alzheimer's—because of a combination of your environment and genes inherited from your parents. The agents that cause infectious disease are called *pathogens* or *parasites*. While biologists once used 'parasite' only to describe relatively large disease-causing agents such as tapeworms or ticks, they now include microorganisms (viruses, bacteria, and fungi) in this category as well, making the two terms more or less synonymous.

Infectious disease frightens us precisely *because* it is infectious. Its agents are usually invisible to the naked eye and thus largely unavoidable, except by entirely eschewing human contact. Edgar Allan Poe illustrated the fear of infection, as well as the futility of cutting off human contact to evade infectious disease, in his 1842 story *The Masque of the Red Death*. In Poe's story, a group of wealthy nobles withdraw to an isolated location to escape from a plague called the Red Death. Ultimately, a costumed stranger infiltrates the group at a masquerade ball. Despite their precautions, the entire group succumbs to the disease.

However ineffective it might be, for most of human history the strategy taken by Poe's nobles—avoiding disease transmission—has been the only way to combat infectious disease. Since the mechanisms of disease transmission were unknown until the mid-19th century, all human societies could do in the face of an epidemic was to cut off contact with infected areas. In 1665, Isaac Newton retreated to the countryside to avoid the Great Plague of London—and incidentally invented calculus and discovered the law of gravity. In the same year, the English village of Eyam voluntarily quarantined itself to prevent the spread of the plague, with half or more of the villagers ultimately dying. The word 'quarantine', which now describes the compulsory isolation of potentially infected people to avoid transmission to others, is derived from the forty days that ships had to wait outside the city of Venice to be sure they were free of plague.

Quarantines (at least those better than the one in Poe's story) do block transmission, but they are fundamentally reactive—they are only imposed once we become aware of a serious threat of disease. They help only healthy people living in uninfected populations, not individuals who have already been infected or uninfected people unlucky enough to be stuck in the quarantine zone. On the other hand, quarantines can be effective against any disease, provided that we know something about its mode of transmission (since plague is spread by rat fleas, preventing communication among humans while allowing rats to move freely is useless).

Quarantines are deployed to protect groups of people, rather than individuals. As medical science improved, public health officials began to shift their focus from the protection of populations to the protection of individuals. Immunization—the process of protecting people by stimulating their immune systems with foreign substances such as mild pathogen strains or toxins—was the first of several major breakthroughs in individual-focused infectious disease control. Immunization for smallpox was widely practised in Africa, China, India, and Turkey by the early 18th century. It achieved public visibility in the West following its importation to England in 1721 by Lady Mary Wortley Montagu, the wife of the British ambassador to Turkey, and more spectacularly via an 'experiment' in the same year promoted by clergyman Cotton Mather of the colonial city of Boston, Massachusetts. In the face of a smallpox outbreak, Mather and his medical colleague Zabdiel Boylston promoted immunization rather recklessly, against the will of the majority of his fellow Bostonians. Despite several deaths, the experiment demonstrated an effective alternative to physical isolation: immunization protected individuals from infection without restricting anyone's freedom of movement.

Mather and Boylston's experiment also illustrated an ethical conflict between controlling disease for the benefit of an individual and controlling disease for the benefit of an entire population. Bostonians who were successfully immunized were safe from disease, but for several days following immunization they could have transmitted the disease to unprotected individuals. Most modern immunizations involve non-infectious substances, so this particular problem is of lesser concern today, but the conflict between individual and public health is very much alive.

Most immunizations can only prevent healthy individuals from becoming infected, not cure infected people. Individual-level control of disease took another leap forward in the mid-20th century with the advent of antibiotic chemicals. First derived from common household moulds and bacteria and later synthesized in the laboratory, antibiotics could be used to cure individuals who were already infected. The possibility of curing disease also lessened the fear of quarantine, which had previously been seen as a death sentence.

Between antibiotics to cure harmful bacterial infections and a wave of new and effective vaccines to prevent diseases such as polio, measles, and pertussis, an infectious disease-free future must have seemed within reach to the public health officials of the 1970s. However, public health officials were quickly faced with proof that individual-level control fails for many diseases. Vaccines work by priming the human immune system, and thus they are much harder to develop for disease agents such as malaria or HIV that have evolved strategies for evading the immune system. Antibiotics are only effective against bacteria, not other microorganisms such as viruses or fungi (while antiviral and antifungal chemicals do exist, they are much less broadly effective than antibiotics). With the realization in the late 20th century that infectious diseases were not vanquished after all, research began to shift back towards population-level control.

So far we have divided treatments according to whether they primarily help populations (quarantine) or individuals (immunization/vaccination, antibiotics). Looking more closely, however, we can see that both antibiotics and immunization do help protect populations, as well as benefiting the individuals who receive treatment. Using drugs to cure sick people reduces the impact of infectious disease, because people who recover also stop infecting others. Thus, treating sick people can reduce transmission. Using vaccines to protect people from infection means that some potentially infectious contacts (activities by infected people such as sneezing or sexual activity, depending on the disease) are wasted on people who are protected from disease, again reducing transmission. This so-called *herd immunity* reduces the size of an epidemic even beyond the direct effects of vaccination. If we immunize enough of the population, we can reduce transmission sufficiently to stamp out an epidemic. If we can do this at a global scale, then the disease will become extinct (as in the case of smallpox, one extinction that environmentalists don't worry about).

If the problem were just that some diseases are harder to control than others, we would still be making progress, albeit slowly, in the fight against infectious disease. Modern molecular biology has provided us with a variety of new antiviral drugs, and vaccines are in development even for such difficult cases as malaria. But both humans and infectious disease agents are living organisms, and all living organisms undergo ecological and evolutionary change, making infectious disease a moving target. Our growing recognition that we (and our plagues!) are tied to the wheel of life, and our realization that individual-level approaches have failed to free us from the wheel, drives the shift in infectious disease research today.

Ecological processes

As much as we try to deny it, humans are subject to the laws of ecology. We control most aspects of our environment. Motor vehicles have replaced large predators as the leading category of violent death; we have wiped out most of our potential competitors; and we have domesticated the organisms below us on the food chain. But infectious disease still connects us to the global web of life.

The most important disease–ecology connection is *zoonosis*, the transmission of new diseases from animal *reservoir hosts* to humans: Ebola (probably from bats) may be the most spectacular example, but many of the new and emerging diseases that we haven't got a handle on come from animals: SARS, avian (H5N1) influenza, and hantavirus are a few of the better-known examples. In fact, almost all infectious diseases originate in this way, and the majority of emerging disease threats are zoonotic. Since it is difficult to vaccinate or design drugs against unknown diseases, this parade of new threats is terrifying: we don't know when a 'super-disease' might emerge.

Zoonoses are by no means new. Smallpox is thought to have moved from rodents into humans at least 16,000 years ago; measles moved from cattle to humans sometime around the 9th century; and HIV jumped from monkeys and chimpanzees to humans in the early 20th century. However, rapid human population growth and changes in land use have increased human–animal contact, whether in the tropical rainforest (HIV and Ebola) or in the temperate suburbs (Lyme disease).

As well as coming into more contact with animals, humans are moving around the planet at an accelerating pace. Contact between individuals, and thus transmission, can happen much faster and over much greater distances than when Isaac Newton escaped the plague in the 17th century or when Poe penned *The Masque of the Red Death* in the 19th century. Diseases that had previously been confined to narrow regions (generally developing countries) can rapidly expand their ranges. This is true not only for human infectious diseases, but also for diseases affecting other species whose infectious agents are transported by humans in our luggage, in the food with which we sustain ourselves during travel, or on our shoes. Human travel and commerce can spread disease indirectly, by transporting *vectors*: animals (especially insects) that transmit disease from one organism to another. For example, the international trade in used tyres is spreading *Aedes* mosquitoes, the vector of dengue fever. As well as vectors, we sometimes move the reservoir hosts of zoonoses. The first human infections of the Ebola virus outside of Africa, in 1989, came from monkeys (crab-eating macaques) that had been imported from the Philippines for animal experimentation: luckily, the particular strain involved (Ebola Reston) turned out to be harmless to humans.

Increasing movement spreads vectors and hosts to new areas; environmental change allows them to thrive in their new homes. With global climate change, animals and especially temperature-sensitive insects can invade new areas in temperate regions. Although the topic is still controversial, many climate scientists and some epidemiologists are convinced that mosquito-borne diseases like dengue and malaria are already spreading to new populations under the influence of regional climate change. An even greater impact comes from more localized environmental changes driven by human patterns of settlement and economic activity. For example, the larvae of dengue-transmitting mosquitoes thrive in water bodies as small as used tyres and household water tanks. More generally, as people in the developing world move from rural to ever-growing urban environments, they face greater sewage problems (spreading cholera and other water-borne disease) and encounter new and different kinds of disease-bearing insects.

Evolutionary processes

Ecology constantly exposes us to new epidemics, but evolution is even worse: the diseases we already know change even as we attempt to come to grips with them. As living organisms fighting for survival, infectious diseases don't accidentally escape our attempts to control them. They are actually driven by natural selection to escape. Infectious disease is a moving target that moves faster the harder we try to hit it. Disease biologists frequently invoke Lewis Carroll's Red Queen from *Through the Looking Glass*, who says: 'it takes all the running you can do, to keep in the same place'.

For every disease prevention strategy, infectious diseases have an evolutionary countermeasure. Bacteria did not evolve antibiotic resistance in response to human antibiotic use: scientists have found antibiotic resistance genes similar to modern variants in DNA extracted from 30,000-year-old frozen soil. This isn't surprising, because humans did not invent antibiotics. Rather, we borrowed or coopted them from fungi, which had evolved them as a strategy for combating bacteria. However, the widespread use of antibiotics in both medicine and agriculture has allowed bacteria that are resistant to one or more types of antibiotic to outcompete their susceptible counterparts. Other organisms, such as the protozoans that cause malaria, have also evolved resistance to the drugs used to treat them. And when HIV patients are given a single drug rather than a multi-drug 'cocktail', the virus evolves drug resistance within their bodies in just a few weeks. Pathogens evolve resistance to vaccines as well as drugs, but in a different way. Rather than resistance genes spreading within the pathogen population, *strain replacement* occurs—previously rare types that are immune to our vaccines take over the population.

Although mosquitoes have smaller populations and lower birth rates than bacteria and viruses, and hence evolve much more slowly, they too have found evolutionary countermeasures to our disease control strategies. In the developed world, DDT use was discontinued as Rachel Carson and others spread the alarm about its harmful effects on wildlife, but vector control strategies based on DDT were short-lived even in developing countries because

DDT-resistant mosquitoes evolved within a decade of the onset of mass spraying programmes.

Every aspect of infectious disease biology, not just the ability to resist or circumvent control measures, is constantly evolving. Biologists have noted that the virulence of a disease—how harmful it is to its host—is an evolutionary characteristic of the pathogenic organism. Typically mild diseases can suddenly acquire a mutation that makes them much nastier. A single mutation in the West Nile virus (WNV) that arose in the late 1990s made it far more lethal to crows, although we don't know whether the same mutation is also associated with increased virulence of WNV in humans.

Although mutations are random, evolution by natural selection is not: once pathogens mutate, their subsequent success depends on ecological conditions. Biologist Paul Ewald was among the first to point out that changes in pathogens' ecological conditions, such as a shift from direct person-to-person transmission to water-borne transmission, could favour more virulent forms of infectious diseases. The rise of global air travel may drive evolutionary as well as ecological changes in disease: some biologists have pointed out that mixing between spatially separated populations can encourage virulence.

Outlook

Given these challenges, the elimination of infectious disease—the siren song of the 20th century—seems hopelessly naïve, and approaches based solely on protecting individuals appear untenable. It would seem that we must learn to live with infectious disease, rather than eliminate it. However, we must also strive to reduce the misery caused by infectious disease. Accordingly, this century has seen a shift from attempts to eliminate the agents of infectious disease, to attempts to understand, predict, and manage infectious disease transmission at the population level. The primary tools in this new theoretical effort are not technologies of magic bullets, but instead the disciplines of ecology and evolution. Ecology, because understanding ecological relationships helps us understand cycles of transmission. Evolution, because disease agents evolve, both on their own and in response to our efforts to control them.

Chapter 2
Transmission at different scales

Transmission defines infectious disease. Transmission occurs when someone passes a disease to someone else: technically speaking, when a pathogen that was established in one host organism's body succeeds in moving into another host's body and establishing itself there.

Transmission occurs in a huge variety of ways. For example, in transmission of influenza (a respiratory disease), virus particles produced by the cells in an infected person's lungs would first be coughed or sneezed into the surrounding atmosphere. The infectious particles can survive briefly in the air or on surfaces in the environment, and thus be directly transmitted from person to person with minimal contact. The receiving person could either inhale them directly, or could pick them up by touching a surface shortly after virus-containing droplets landed there. The receiver would then transfer virus particles to their nose by touching their face; from there, the natural movement of air within their nose would move the virus into their respiratory tract. In the respiratory tract, the virus particles would enter vulnerable cells and resume their cycle of spreading from one cell to another within the host's body.

Many viruses, including influenza and diarrhoea-causing viruses such as rotavirus, can survive for days in the environment, building up on particular kinds of objects known as *fomites*. Have you noticed a sudden increase in male physicians sporting bow ties? This fashion statement is a response to health researchers' identification of standard ties as fomites. Influenza viruses can even survive for several days on banknotes, especially if they are first mixed with 'nasopharyngeal secretions' (snot), although we don't actually know whether this transmission pathway is important in real epidemics.

Pathogens whose infectious particles die almost instantaneously outside the warm, wet environment of the human body often rely on bodily fluids being directly transferred from person to person, as in the case of sexually transmitted diseases such as HIV (see Chapter 4) and gonorrhoea. While sexual contact was the most common form of fluid exchange throughout most of human evolutionary history, these pathogens can also be transmitted by more modern modes of fluid exchange such as blood transfusions or the sharing of syringes by drug users.

Other pathogens that cannot survive in the environment have evolved to use other organisms, especially blood-sucking insects and mites, as *vectors* to travel from one host to another. This strategy requires considerably more biological machinery than direct transfer between the bodies of two hosts of the same species. In the extreme case of pathogens with complex life cycles such as malaria (see Chapter 6), the pathogen goes through major transformations within the body of the mosquito vector. In fact, from the perspective of a mosquito-inhabiting malaria parasite, a human is just a convenient way to transmit itself to another mosquito.

Other infectious diseases can persist much better outside of the hosts' bodies. Diseases such as cholera (see Chapter 5), typhoid, and Legionnaires' disease can survive in water, making their way from one host to another through drinking water or air conditioning systems. Anthrax—which kills its hosts quickly, reducing the potential for direct transmission from one animal host to another—produces long-lasting spores that survive for years in the environment, infecting grazing animals years later when they ingest spores attached to soil particles. Many fungi, such as certain species of *Aspergillus*, live primarily as free-living organisms, but can sometimes grow within human hosts if they find themselves there, especially if the host has its immune system weakened by stress or infection with other diseases. (These are called *opportunistic* infectious diseases, in contrast to the *obligate* dependence of most pathogens. Opportunistic infections can live in a host if one is available, but do not require a host in order to complete their life cycles.) The amphibian fungus *Batrachochytrium dendrobatidis* (Chapter 7) is closely related to non-pathogenic soil-dwelling fungi, but is itself an obligate parasite—as far as we know it can only persist in the environment for a few weeks.

Filters for encounter and compatibility

Following the work of Claude Combes, we can break the process of transmission down into three stages: (1) transfer of infectious particles from inside the original host's body to the environment; (2) transfer of infectious particles through the environment, or through the bodies of intermediary vectors or hosts, to the receiving host; (3) transfer of particles from the environment into parts of the receiving host's body such as the blood, lungs, or liver where the pathogen can reproduce. These three stages collectively comprise the *encounter filter*.

Having made it into a new host's body, the travelling pathogen must overcome physical, biochemical, and immunological barriers in order to grow in the body of the new host. In other words, even if the pathogen can pass the encounter filter, it must also be biologically compatible with the new host; this final stage is called the *compatibility filter*. A host could close its compatibility filter by having a disease-resistant genetic mutation, such as the sickle-cell variant of the haemoglobin gene that protects against malaria. Opportunistic fungal infections are usually blocked as long as the host has a properly functioning immune system. In order to block most viral diseases, however, the host's immune system needs to have encountered the pathogen before, either naturally or through vaccination.

Both the encounter and compatibility filters must be open in order for successful transmission to occur. Public health measures can close the encounter filter and are especially important in the early stages of an epidemic. Drugs or vaccines can close the compatibility filter, but they are not always available.

Methods for closing the encounter filter include simple preventive strategies such as quarantine (see Chapter 1). They also include environmental strategies such as improved sanitation to control water-borne disease, or mosquito and tick control to stop vector-borne disease. Another class of strategies tries to convince people to modify their behaviour. These include the US Centers for Disease Control and Prevention's advice to 'Cover Your Cough' to stop influenza, as well as their suggestions for avoiding mosquito-borne diseases such as West Nile virus: stay indoors at dusk, wear long pants and long-sleeved shirts, and use insect repellent. Though changing people's behaviour is difficult, it is usually the cheapest way to control disease. You don't need to inject or swallow substances that may have harmful side effects, and behavioural changes can even protect against unknown pathogens. Avoiding exchanging bodily fluids with strangers is a good idea, even if they have been screened for all currently known diseases.

Epidemic dynamics

It's easy to understand the encounter and compatibility filters at the individual level: if you can prevent the transfer of infectious particles from the environment into your body, or if you immunize yourself to prevent the infection from taking hold in your body, you can stay safe. In order to understand the effects of these filters at the population level—for example, to decide whether an immunization programme or a quarantine will stop an epidemic—we need mathematical models. Almost as soon as biologists began to understand the mechanics of disease transmission, mathematicians started to develop models to describe the effects of the encounter and compatibility filters at the population level. As early as 1760, Daniel Bernoulli, a member of an eminent Swiss family of mathematicians and scientists, used a mathematical model to describe to what extent smallpox immunization (i.e. closing the compatibility filter for some individuals) could improve public health. Bernoulli concluded that immunization could increase the expected lifespan at birth by 10 per cent, from about twenty-seven to thirty years (the expected lifespan at birth was very short in the 18th century because of the high rate of infant and childhood mortality).

Bernoulli's model only took into account the direct benefits of immunization, thus missing the key insight of herd immunity. Immunization protects the people who are immunized, but it also reduces the prevalence of the disease and thus provides an indirect benefit to non-immunized people. To eradicate disease, you don't need to close the compatibility and encounter filters entirely (i.e. immunize 100 per cent of the people, or prevent transmission 100 per cent of the time); you just need to reduce transmission enough so that each infectious case gives rise to less than one new case. In technical terms, you need to reduce the *reproductive number*—the average number of new cases generated by a single case—to less than 1. If you succeed, then the disease will die out in the population as a whole, even if a few unlucky people still get infected.

The reproductive number depends on the biology of the disease: how quickly can it produce new infectious particles? How well do they survive in the environment? It also depends on the ecology and behaviour of the host, which controls the encounter filter: how dense is the population, how do hosts interact with each other, and how often do they interact? Finally, it depends on the fraction of the population that remains susceptible to the disease, which declines over the course of an epidemic as individuals first get infected and then recover (typically becoming immune, at least temporarily) or die. To ignore this last complication, epidemiologists focus on the *intrinsic reproductive number*, R_0 (pronounced 'R-zero' or 'R-nought'), which is the number of cases that would be generated by the first case in a new outbreak. R_0 is a basic measure of disease biology and community structure; it doesn't depend on how far the epidemic has spread through the population. If you can close the compatibility and encounter filters far enough to reduce the intrinsic reproductive number to less than 1, then you can not only control an epidemic in progress, but prevent the disease from getting started in the first place.

The importance of this kind of average-centred, population-level thinking in disease control was first appreciated by Ronald Ross, who built mathematical models of malaria transmission to prove that malaria could be eradicated without completely eliminating mosquitoes, by reducing mosquito populations below a threshold level—so that on average each infected human led to less than one new human case. (As we will see in Chapter 6, mosquito control and other methods for closing the encounter and compatibility filters have successfully eradicated malaria in some places, but not worldwide.) Ross won the Nobel Prize in 1902 for elucidating the life cycle of malaria, but his biography at the Nobel Foundation's website states that 'perhaps his greatest [contribution] was the development of mathematical models for the study of [malaria] epidemiology'.

Ross's model was one of the first *compartmental models*, which divide the population into compartments according to their disease status and track the rates at which individuals change from one disease status to another. The most common, simplest compartmental model is called the *SIR model* because it divides the population up into *Susceptible*, *Infective*, and *Recovered* people. Susceptibles are people who could get infected, but are not currently infected (i.e. their compatibility filter is open); infectives have the disease and can transmit it (i.e. they are *infectious* as well as infected); recovered people have had the disease and are at least temporarily immune.

The original compartmental models spawned many variations: for example, SIS models represent diseases such as gonorrhoea where individuals go straight back into the susceptible compartment once they have been cured of disease (say by taking antibiotics), because there is no effective immunity. Dozens of books and thousands of scientific papers have been written about compartmental models. Although the original versions were very simple, researchers have since added all kinds of complexity, accounting for the effects of genetics, age, and nutrition on the compatibility filter, and constructing various representations of social and spatial networks to model the encounter filter. Compartmental models also form the basic structure of huge computer models that track the behaviour and infection status of every individual in the US population in order to understand the spatial spread of influenza epidemics.

While realism and faithfulness to the biological facts of a given disease are important, compartmental models have remained the workhorse of epidemiological modelling because, even in their simpler forms, they capture most of the important characteristics of the spread of disease through a population. Especially when we are ignorant of important information about a disease—a situation painfully familiar to epidemiologists—an oversimplified model can be more useful than an overcomplicated one, as long as we interpret its conclusions cautiously.

Compartmental models typically assume that everyone in the population starts out equally susceptible to a particular disease (at birth, or in the case of sexually transmitted diseases, once they become sexually active). Susceptibles get infected by mixing with infected people in some way—for example, being coughed or sneezed on or exchanging bodily fluids. In general the infection rate increases with the proportion of infected people in the population, but the details vary enormously among models. After an *infectious period* during which they spread disease, infected people recover; they move into the recovered compartment and gain effective immunity to the disease. As we have seen, a huge number of variations on this model are possible, including subdividing the population by age, sex, or geographic location; allowing people to return to the susceptible class from the recovered class after some time period; or allowing for variation in the rate at which different individuals transmit disease.

Even without going into any of the underlying mathematics, the structure of the SIR model (Figure 1) helps categorize the ways we can control epidemics. The most common control strategy—closing the compatibility filter by immunization or *prophylactic* drug treatment (i.e. giving people drugs to prevent rather than cure disease)—moves individuals directly from the susceptible to the recovered compartment without passing through the infected compartment on the way. Almost all other epidemic control measures affect the encounter filter in one way or another. For epidemics in wildlife or domestic animals and plants, killing susceptible or infected individuals (*culling*) removes these individuals from the population entirely, hopefully reducing R_0 below 1. Culling is one of the few available strategies, albeit a very controversial one, for controlling the foot and mouth disease virus in cattle. Post-exposure treatment increases the rate at which individuals move into the recovered compartment, importantly shortening their infectious period and reducing the number of susceptibles they can infect. Finally, transmission controls such as quarantines block infection without moving individuals between compartments.

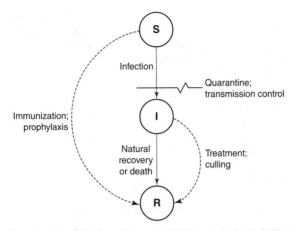

1. The SIR model describes the progression of people through disease stages from susceptible to infectious to recovered. Interventions such as culling, treatment, or quarantine can speed up or prevent transition among compartments.

As well as a conceptual framework for thinking about disease control measures, the SIR model also provides a quantitative framework for calculating exactly how much control is necessary to eradicate a disease, or how much a given level of control will reduce the level of disease in the population. Suppose we can eliminate some fraction of effective contacts, by a *control fraction* (p), by closing either the compatibility filter (e.g. by vaccination) or the encounter filter (e.g. by providing condoms or clean needles). Then the value of R_0 will be reduced by a factor $1 - p$; if R_0 is initially equal to 4 and we can achieve a control fraction of 0.75 or 75 per cent, then we will reduce R_0 to $(1 - 0.75) \times 4 = 1$.

A little bit of algebra shows that in order to reduce R_0 to less than 1 we need to increase the control above a critical value of $p_{crit} = 1 - 1/R_0$ (Figure 2). This tells us immediately why it was much easier to eliminate smallpox ($R_0 \approx 6$, $p_{crit} \approx 0.8$) than it has been to eliminate measles ($R_0 \approx 15$, $p_{crit} \approx 0.95$), despite the fact that cheap and effective vaccines are available for both diseases,

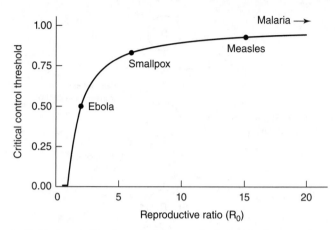

2. Critical control level required (proportion immunized or treated to prevent transmission) to eradicate an infectious disease, based on its R_0 value.

and why it will be extremely difficult to eradicate malaria, even once we have an effective vaccine: R_0 is estimated to be greater than 100 in some areas, so the critical control fraction will be greater than 99 per cent. In fact, the only way to eradicate malaria in high-disease areas will likely be to combine several different strategies (e.g. vaccine and mosquito control), each of which could have (say) 90 per cent effectiveness, so that their combined efficacy could reach the 99 per cent level that might be required.

In principle, if disease control measures can reduce R_0 below 1, they will not only terminate any existing epidemic, but will prevent recurrence of the epidemic as long as the control measures are maintained. Eradicating a disease within a given region, such as the UK or Europe, reduces the local burden of infectious disease, but does not eliminate the need for disease control unless public health authorities can somehow be 100 per cent sure that they can prevent the importation of disease from outside the eradication zone. Only if we can eradicate a disease globally, as has so far been done only for smallpox and rinderpest (a lethal cattle disease closely related to measles), can control measures safely be discontinued. This makes eradicating a disease, rather than simply controlling it, an attractive policy option—once the disease is completely gone, any resources that went into managing it can be freed for other disease control efforts, or for other societal goals.

Of course, knowing R_0 does not tell us everything about controlling disease—diseases such as influenza ($R_0 \approx 2 - 3$) and HIV ($R_0 \approx 2 - 5$) are harder to control than their relatively low R_0 values would suggest. Sometimes treatments are unavailable, or too expensive. In other cases, treatment or control measures are only partly effective. With a vaccine that is only 50 per cent effective, comparable to the experimental malaria vaccines currently being tested, and better than the best HIV vaccines available (≈ 30 per cent effective), twice as many people need to be treated (if $R_0 > 2$ it would be impossible to eradicate the disease with this vaccine). Another problem is that infections may be hard to detect, and thus be out of reach of disease control efforts, for either biological or cultural reasons. Biologically, some individuals (carriers) can be infected and spread a disease while showing no symptoms; culturally, many diseases carry a stigma that makes people hide the fact that they are infected. During the ongoing West African Ebola epidemic, one of the major concerns about imposing harsh control measures is that they may simply encourage people exposed to Ebola to hide from authorities.

Compartmental models tell us much more than the level of control necessary to eradicate disease locally or globally. They also give a simple formula for the number of people who will be affected by a disease outbreak in the absence of control, or the size of the susceptible population at equilibrium for a disease that becomes established in the population. Compartmental models have also helped epidemiologists to think about the dynamics of disease—the ways that the infected population changes over time.

For example, one of the first applications of compartmental models explained that observed multi-year cycles of measles epidemics did not necessarily mean that a new genetic type was invading every few years; rather, disease spread so fast that the susceptible population was exhausted and required several years to build up to the point where it could support another major outbreak. Similarly, mathematicians have pointed out that vaccination campaigns that fail to eradicate a disease allow the number of susceptibles in the population to build up. Even if vaccination coverage stays high, these build-ups may lead to large outbreaks several years after the beginning of the campaign. Without this dynamical insight, the outbreak could easily be interpreted as a sudden change in the effectiveness of the vaccine or the transmissibility of the disease, rather than as a straightforward consequence of a sub-critical level of control.

Within-host disease dynamics

One of the many biological details that compartmental models omit in their quest for simplicity is any description of the way that disease plays out within an individual host. In compartmental models, hosts are either infected or not; we don't keep track of the level of infection within an individual (e.g. the number of virus-infected cells or the density of the virus in the bloodstream), nor of the response of the individual's immune system to the disease.

Standard compartmental models are best for understanding small pathogens (*microparasites*) such as viruses, bacteria, and fungi; because these types of pathogens tend to build up very quickly within a host, and trigger similar immune responses in most hosts, characterizing hosts as either infected or uninfected is a reasonable simplification. In populations infected with *macroparasites*—larger parasites such as tapeworms or ticks—the number of parasites per host varies greatly among individuals.

To account for this variation, mathematicians have had to design more complex models. Within the last decade or so, however, these distinctions have begun to blur as researchers build more elaborate microparasite models that track changes in the numbers of infected particles or cells and the level of activation of the immune system within an individual. For example, a large fraction of HIV transmission occurs within the first month of infection. If we want to understand and predict HIV epidemics, we obviously need to use models that distinguish between recently- and not-so-recently-infected people; we might even want to track the precise level of virus in the blood and other bodily fluids of an infected person.

Nested models, which track both changes in the number of infected people and changes in the number of infected cells within individuals, are mathematically complex—one can imagine the difficulty of keeping track of all of the virus particles within every individual in a population! Somewhat more manageable are within-host models, which focus on the progress of disease within a typical person, ignoring how the disease is spreading among individuals. Where epidemiological models represent the progress of disease in a population, and give insight into the impact and control of disease at the population level, within-host models can help understand how disease works within a single individual.

Despite this difference in scope, however, epidemiological models and within-host models have striking similarities (Figure 3). The compartmental model can easily be adapted for within-host models, especially for parasites such as viruses that must invade host cells in order to reproduce. Instead of assuming that infection builds up quickly and characteristically within individual hosts so that we can practically treat them as either uninfected or infected, we now assume that the level of infection (e.g. the number of virus particles) builds up quickly and characteristically within host *cells*. The concepts of encounter and compatibility filters are just as useful on the within-host as the within-population levels,

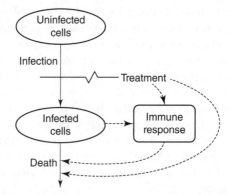

3. A within-host compartmental model showing: the infection of cells and death of infected cells; triggering of the immune response by infected cells and by treatment; killing of infected cells by the immune response and by treatment; and blocking of between-cell transmission by treatment.

describing how infection gets from one cell to another and what prevents or allows infection of a cell by a disease particle.

Within-host models often add a new compartment to keep track of free-floating infectious particles outside of cells, and they often include a separate term for the level of immune defences activated within a host. Within-host models usually assume that the strength of immune defences increases as the number of infected cells increases. If the immune response is rapid enough and strong enough, these models show how the immune system can naturally overwhelm an infection, although not necessarily before the infection has had time to proliferate temporarily and infect another host. Within-host models can also show how drug treatments can slow down disease spread within the host sufficiently for the immune response to eradicate the disease. In viruses such as HIV and the human T-lymphotropic virus that attack immune cells, within-host models show exactly how these diseases pervert the normal immune strategy; the immune system responds to the presence of virus infection by activating more immune cells, which in turn provide more resources for virus growth. This is like finding out that you're trying to put out a fire with gasoline instead of water.

Virulence, resistance, and tolerance

Compartmental models have been used most often for widespread diseases where nearly everyone in the population is equally susceptible, such as measles, polio, or smallpox. Humans do vary in their susceptibility to infection: because they have different genotypes (i.e. complete sets of genetic material), or are better or worse nourished, or are more or less stressed. They also vary in infectiousness, how badly they suffer, and how likely they are to die from the disease. However, for the purposes of epidemiological planning it's often wise to ignore these details, at least initially.

When we turn to thinking about evolution, this variation becomes not just dangerous to ignore, but central to the questions we are asking. In the last few decades, epidemiological modellers have turned from just trying to understand how diseases spread in populations over timescales from days to years, to trying to understand how diseases evolve over timescales from years to thousands of years. What is it about the combination of a particular host, a particular parasite, and a particular environment that allows the parasite to infect a host? What determines whether the host is badly harmed by the infection or only has mild symptoms?

We have to make several important distinctions about the characteristics of parasites. The first is between infectiousness (how easily the parasite can infect the host) and virulence (how severely it affects the host if it succeeds). We often treat infectiousness and virulence as fixed properties of a parasite. Smallpox has much more horrible symptoms than measles, and a much higher chance of killing the host, regardless of the particular genetic makeup of the parasite or of the host it infects. Measles is always more infectious than smallpox, which is more infectious than HIV or Ebola. In principle, however, we can imagine two parasite strains and two kinds of hosts that 'cross over' in their effects, with one parasite having higher virulence on the first host genotype than the second and the other having higher virulence on the second genotype.

Hosts could control the infectivity and virulence of the pathogens attacking them in two ways. If the host is able to close the compatibility filter partially or completely, we say that it *resists* the parasite. As a result the parasite might not be able to infect the host at all, or it might not be able to build up its population within the host to very high levels, so that the host suffers few ill effects. Alternatively, the host might allow the parasite to infect it (or more precisely it might not invest energy in defending itself), but it could evolve mechanisms so that it was not badly harmed by infection: in this case, we would call the host tolerant rather than resistant.

Tolerance and resistance have similar outcomes at the level of the individual host (the host isn't harmed by the parasite), but very different outcomes at the level of the population. If some individuals are highly susceptible (neither resistant nor tolerant), then the presence of resistant individuals will help them by lowering the overall chances of infection, while tolerant individuals will increase the chance of infection. This is one reason that epidemiologists worry about the introduction of partially effective vaccines. If pathogens evolved to replicate more quickly within the host in order to overcome partial resistance in vaccinated people, they might increase their virulence in non-vaccinated people; if vaccination makes people tolerant rather than resistant to disease, they could still spread infection to unvaccinated people.

Chapter 3
Influenza

Unless you are lucky or very careful, you have probably had influenza (the flu) sometime in your life. Flu is familiar to almost everyone, occurring in every country, every year. It has been with us throughout history. Though not as gruesome as some viral diseases such as Ebola, the flu virus has caused more deaths than any single disease outbreak since the Black Death (bubonic plague) of the 14th century: twenty to fifty million people worldwide died from the 1918 Spanish Flu.

Furthermore, although non-epidemiologists may not think of it as a big problem, the annual flu epidemic that occurs every winter in temperate parts of the world infects millions of people. Although influenza kills only a small fraction of even the frailest elderly population, it is still thought to cause as many as 40,000 deaths in the US in a typical year (not a pandemic year). Because influenza causes many deaths indirectly, e.g. due to secondary infections, these numbers are estimated indirectly by estimating how many extra deaths are observed in years with large seasonal epidemics.

Influenza is even scarier in years, such as 2009, when we think we might be on the verge of a deadly pandemic that could cause millions rather than tens of thousands of deaths. Pandemics arise under very particular circumstances, but the two most important ingredients are lack of existing immunity (an opening in the compatibility filter) and virulence. If the virus has radically changed its appearance, more people than average will be susceptible because their immunity from previous years fails to protect them against the new strain. This drives the value of R_0 (the intrinsic reproductive rate, see Chapter 2) higher than in a typical year. Higher transmission is scariest if the virus is simultaneously more virulent, severely harming a larger fraction of its victims than usual. Authorities feared this situation in 2009 for three reasons: (1) the new strain was of the H1N1 type, different from the previous year's H3N2 type, which would lead to more susceptibility and a higher R_0; (2) the highly virulent 1918 pandemic was caused by an H1N1 strain; (3) the 2009 strain's virulence was initially overestimated due to biases in reporting from its origin in Mexico.

In the end the 2009 strain's virulence turned out to be about average for a flu strain overall, although it did affect younger people relatively severely, leading to more years of life lost. The 2009 H1N1 strain did officially lead to a pandemic—that is, it was a previously unobserved strain that caused significant numbers of cases all over the world—but happily it did not infect as many people, nor kill as many of them, as initially feared.

In order to prevent pandemics, we have to control transmission. Transmission can be controlled by reducing encounters (sneezing into your elbow instead of into your hand), by reducing compatibility (vaccinating to reduce the number of susceptible individuals), or ideally by a combination of both. In the 2009 H1N1 epidemic, encounter rates were reduced by closing schools throughout Mexico, as well as by discouraging large public gatherings and distributing masks and hand sanitizer. Development of a vaccine to close the compatibility filter for the new strain was swift; the vaccine became available in October 2009, a mere six months after the strain was characterized. Vaccines were initially limited, so were first distributed to the target groups believed to be most at risk, *and* to those most likely to transmit the disease, including school-age children. We'll come back to why children are an important target group for flu vaccination later in this chapter.

In first-world countries, the flu shot (or at least the ubiquitous publicity surrounding the vaccine) is as much a harbinger of winter as the shortening of the days. Unlike the measles or diphtheria vaccines that we in the developed world get once as children, we need new flu shots every year because the flu virus evolves rapidly; it changes its outer garments so fast that our immune system needs new clues each year to recognize the current disguise of this old and otherwise familiar foe.

To understand flu control, it helps to understand the evolutionary processes that lead to flu's unique capacity for costume changes. As discussed in Chapter 1, hosts and parasites are like Alice and the Red Queen in *Through the Looking Glass*: they have to run as fast as they can to stay in the same place. Hosts and parasites are locked in a race, with the host evolving to escape the parasite and the parasite counter-evolving to keep up with the host. For the host, winning the race means closing the compatibility filter so that the parasite can no longer exploit it. For the parasite, winning means keeping the compatibility filter open, so it can continue to exploit the host. Thus, 'the same place' means the parasite can still infect the host; running as fast as they can means both the host and parasite are rapidly evolving, with one trying to set itself free and the other stubbornly holding on.

It is important to remember that evolution does not always mean evolution via natural selection, the usual 'survival of the fittest' paradigm that you may remember from school. Any natural population contains organisms with many different genotypes; the current proportion of any given genotype within the population is called the *genotype frequency*. To evolutionary biologists, evolution means *any* change in genotype frequencies over time. Popular discussions of evolution mostly focus on the process of natural selection, the change in the frequencies of genotypes because of differences in fitness—i.e. the expected numbers of offspring and probabilities of survival of each genotype. But genotype frequencies can also change due to chance events, a process referred to as *genetic drift*.

To distinguish further between natural selection and genetic drift, let's consider an imaginary infectious disease. Suppose a mutation happens at random in the host genotype that confers complete resistance to the disease and has no bad side effects. If the disease is common, then the mutation should increase in frequency in the population due to natural selection; people who carry the mutation will have higher fitness in the presence of the disease, and the same fitness in its absence. However, there's a small probability that before the mutation has a chance to increase in frequency, the extended family in which it arose will decide to embark on a trip together—and be tragically wiped out in a bus crash. This is an example of genetic drift: evolution happening because of a chance event that has nothing to do with the infectious disease, the host's fitness, or the mutation itself. One of the reasons that predicting flu epidemics is so difficult even for expert epidemiologists is because flu evolves by genetic drift as well as by natural selection; chance events that happen before the temperate flu season can set the year's flu epidemic off down different, unpredictable tracks.

Evolution requires genetic variation. The ultimate source of genetic variation is mutation, a process at which viruses excel. Another important source of genetic variation is recombination, combining existing genotypes in different ways. The influenza virus takes advantage of both mutation and *reassortment*, a type of recombination. As we will explain, hosts' (i.e. humans') power to evolve by mutation is limited, but we make good use of recombination as a key feature of our immune system. The reason we can recognize so many parasites is not because our genes code a different protein (*antibody*) to recognize each one—our genomes would have to be many times their already huge size. Instead, we reuse the same small pieces of genes in different combinations to create a range of antibodies. These different antibodies recognize specific parts of the costumes, which are known as *antigens*, of many different parasites.

Our genomes are made of DNA that is replicated or copied by a special protein called a *polymerase*. Our DNA polymerase not only copies DNA, it also proofreads the new strand being produced, and can correct many of the errors inevitably made during the copying process. The influenza virus has a genome coded in RNA rather than DNA. It also encodes its own RNA polymerase. However, unlike the polymerase that we produce to replicate our DNA, flu's RNA polymerase cannot proofread to correct replication errors. As a result, replicating flu viruses end up with many more errors—that is, mutations—in the new copies of the genome. The virus arising from the new, mutated RNA genome will have the mutation, and so will its offspring. The result is that mutation rates for flu are 100,000 times greater than our own. Because flu mutates rapidly, it evolves rapidly.

Mutations in influenza lead to *antigenic drift*, a process of slow change in the flu virus over time. Under antigenic drift, our bodies can sometimes use the same set of antibodies to recognize strains of flu that have drifted apart. Their short-sleeved shirts may have changed from stripes to solids to plaids, but they are still recognizable as shirts. The new varieties of influenza that result from antigenic drift then evolve through both natural selection—genotypes that are slightly better than average at evading the existing repertoire of host antibodies will have higher fitness—and genetic drift. Because flu constantly evolves, both vaccinated people and unvaccinated people who contract flu naturally tend to lose their immunity after a few years.

The flu has another evolutionary trick. Its genome is divided into eight discrete segments; it can combine different variants of the segments in new ways to result in viruses with novel properties. When two different variants of the flu virus happen to invade the same cell within a host, they can reassort, trading segments of their genomes with one another to produce an *antigenic shift*. This reassortment results in fast, dramatic costume changes, effectively trading a short-sleeved shirt for a smoking jacket. These changes are hard for our immune systems to recognize, so they open the compatibility filter. As a result, the reassorted offspring have an evolutionary advantage and spread in the population—if they are also good at transmitting themselves to other hosts, overcoming the encounter filter.

Antigenic drift is not usually sufficient to cause a pandemic. The hallmark of pandemic flu is antigenic shift, particularly the reassortment of flu strains found in multiple hosts. For example, the 2009 H1N1 flu arose when different segments from viruses that were adapted to birds, humans, and swine came together in pigs.

The constantly changing costume of the flu virus consists of a protein derived from two separate genes, haemagglutinin (HA) and neuraminidase (NA). Flu strains are named for their variants of each gene: H1N1 combines HA variant #1 with NA variant #1. When a given strain of flu swaps its HA and NA genes for another type, our immune system is less able, and sometimes completely unable, to recognize the flu virus. HA and NA are antigens, the parts of a parasite that our immune system uses to recognize it. They are exposed on the surface of virus particles, where our immune system can detect them as they float in the bloodstream. When viruses infect a cell, they turn the cell into a factory for the production of more viruses; in the case of flu, the new viruses emerge from the cell by 'budding' out, rather than bursting the cell altogether. As part of the budding process, infected cells display HA and NA on their surfaces, triggering the recognition and destruction of the co-opted cells by our immune system.

There are two major types of flu vaccine. The standard flu shot (TIV) is an intramuscular injection of inactivated or 'killed' virus. A newer, less widely used type of vaccine, marketed as FluMist or FluEnz, is a nasal spray of attenuated (weakened) but 'live' virus (LAIV). (We put 'killed' and 'live' in quotes here because the consensus among biologists is that viruses are not living organisms, but the terms 'live' and 'killed' are still commonly used.) Both types contain a mixture of three different strains of virus that are predicted to be common during the upcoming flu season. Sometimes some of the same strains are included in consecutive years, if they are still common, but vaccine developers usually include at least one new strain as well, in the hopes of anticipating antigenic drift or shift.

Both TIV and LAIV trigger a response in our most common type of antibody, immunoglobulin G (IgG). IgG is sensitive to the relatively subtle changes that can occur as a result of drift. In other words, if the injection contained only versions of the virus with stripes, and mutations occur that change the costume to a solid colour, our immune system won't be able to detect the changed virus—let alone more complex changes resulting from antigenic shift, i.e. changing T-shirts to smoking jackets. It is this relatively limited ability of IgG to deal with differences in HA and NA, combined with the continuing process of antigenic drift, that requires us to get a new injection with a newly developed vaccine each year.

LAIV also triggers other parts of our immune system, immunoglobulin A (IgA) and cell-mediated immunity (CMI). IgA is another type of antibody that is present in both blood and mucus. CMI is a particularly intriguing form of immunity, not involving antibodies, which is responsible for killing any of our own cells which have been co-opted and turned into virus factories. By destroying the means of virus production rather than just cleaning up virus particles in the bloodstream (see Figure 3), CMI can potentially be far more efficient than antibody-mediated immunity.

If it is so effective, why isn't LAIV given more widely? There are two major reasons. First, and most important, TIV is more effective in generating an immune response in adults—a strong IgG response is better than a weak or absent IgA/CMI response. Second, people who receive LAIV can *shed* virus (i.e. release it into the environment where it can infect others) for a short period after vaccination. This is risky for people with weak immune systems who come in close contact with recently vaccinated people. LAIV is not recommended for people with weakened immune systems, including pregnant women, people under two or over forty-nine, and people with chronic infections such as HIV.

Modern vaccination programmes try to go beyond protecting individuals to protect the entire population. Vaccines can reduce the severity of the annual flu epidemic in several ways. First, they can prevent infection of the vaccinated person altogether. This clearly means less infection—we protect not only our vaccinated individual, but also anyone she would have transmitted disease to if she had been infected. However, even vaccines that do not completely block infection can reduce subsequent transmission. Adults who have received TIV often recover faster than unvaccinated people even when they are unlucky enough to get the flu. This is good for individuals (they suffer symptoms for a shorter time and may be able to get back to work sooner); it also cuts down on overall infection because they have less chance to transmit to others during their shortened infectious period. Vaccinated people may also shed less virus, and hence be less infectious, during the time the virus is present in their bodies. Finally, vaccinated people help control the epidemic via herd immunity (see Chapter 2): potentially infectious contacts of infected people with vaccinated people are wasted (from the pathogen's point of view), leading to a reduction in R_0. If we can successfully immunize enough people (more than a proportion $1 - 1 / R_0$), then infectious people will generate fewer than one new case each and the virus will go extinct.

It is important to prioritize whom to vaccinate first, particularly if vaccine supplies are limited, as was the case early in the 2009 H1N1 outbreak. Even when there is enough vaccine to go around, it is important for public health agencies to decide whom to target with advertising and outreach. One obvious choice is to concentrate on people who are most at risk of severe disease or death. However, many of these people are vulnerable precisely because they have weakened immune systems, which means that vaccination may not protect them even if they can be convinced to get the shot. Another, complementary approach is to focus on vaccinating the people who are most likely to transmit the virus.

Epidemiologists use contact networks to identify individuals within populations who have high transmission rates. Contact networks focus on the 'encounter' stage of transmission—if an uninfected person doesn't encounter an infected one, transmission won't happen. Figure 4 shows a middle-class family in the US, consisting of two parents, two children, and one grandparent. One parent works outside the home in a small business with three other co-workers, while the other parent has an online business and spends a lot of time working in the local coffee shop with a business partner. The two children, aged five and seven, attend the local elementary school. Each child has ten classmates plus one teacher. The grandparent lives independently but near the family's home, and comes over for dinner several times a week.

Casual interactions like saying hello to people only occasionally result in flu transmission. The most important encounters for flu involve regular physical contact, or opportunities for sneezing on and being sneezed upon. Each such contact, for each member of our core family of four, is shown as a line in the figure. This simplified (but not unrealistic) example shows that the children

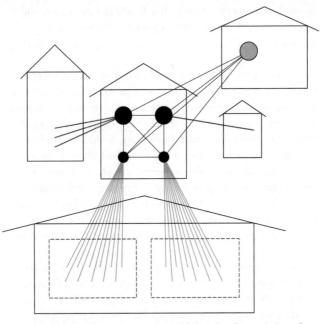

4. Contact network for a Western middle-class family consisting of two parents, two school-age children, and one grandparent living independently.

have the highest number of epidemiologically meaningful encounters. By extension, they are the most likely to bring disease into the family, particularly to the grandparent, who is the most likely to have complications from the flu. For this reason, vaccinating kids is a high priority not only to protect them, but also to protect the elderly. Obviously, contact networks vary considerably from one region to another, as well as by socio-economic status within regions, so careful comparative work is required to set global vaccination priorities.

Flu also represents an interesting case study for an age-old debate: are some kinds of research too dangerous to allow? If people do go ahead and conduct this research, should the results be available only to a limited, carefully screened subset of researchers and policymakers, or should scientific knowledge be available to all?

Scientific research is funded by governmental organizations, non-governmental organizations (NGOs), and industry. Industrial research is usually proprietary—it is kept private so that companies can get a return on their investment. But research funded by governments and NGOs is science for the people. The results of such work should be available to all, particularly when the research is ultimately paid for by taxes and charitable contributions and is directly relevant to human health.

Unfortunately, some of the same research that helps predict pandemics could also be used for nefarious purposes by bioterrorists. Such 'dual-use' research is subject to international treaties and export restrictions. Even if it is not deliberately misused, terrible things could happen if laboratory-developed super-strains accidentally escaped the confines of research labs.

The most critical indicator of pandemic flu—what determines whether a new combination of HA and NA types from avian, porcine, or human sources can spread widely in human populations—is the route of transmission. Flu becomes pandemic only if efficient human-to-human transmission is achieved—specifically, airborne transmission. Thus, an important public health priority is to understand how airborne transmission between humans could evolve and what identifiable hallmarks we should be looking for in order to be able to detect emerging pandemic strains before they spread very far.

Flu research during the first two decades of the 21st century resulted in a face-off between people who embraced the democratization of knowledge and people who feared misuse of that knowledge. The primary motivation behind the controversial research is simple: if we can understand what genetic changes make pandemic flu different from routine seasonal flu, specifically what changes are required to allow airborne transmission, we can potentially see a pandemic strain coming and take appropriate precautions. Maximum response to every case of flu is not an option, because resources are finite and because we value individual freedoms as well as public health. Thus, extraordinary control measures should only be taken when risk is high, but how can we know when that threshold has been crossed?

Flu research became extremely visible in 2011 not because of breakthroughs in understanding pandemics, but because of controversy over the publication of two high-profile papers about airborne transmission. Scientists were studying how H5N1, a particularly virulent strain of avian flu, could achieve airborne transmission from one ferret to another. Ferrets are an important model animal system for studying flu transmission in humans, in part because, like people, ferrets sneeze when they are infected with flu.

The road to publication of this research was long and rocky. The papers were originally submitted in August of 2011. Four months later, the US National Security Advisory Board for Biosecurity initially recommended that key details of the experiments be omitted from the two papers to address security concerns. In May of 2012, the first paper was finally published online, having languished for two months following acceptance. The second paper came out in late June of the same year, and was pithily referred to by *This Week in Virology*, a popular podcast, as 'the second ferret of the apocalypse'. The path to uncensored publication was cleared once experts around the world decided that the potential public health benefits of publication, with all the details, outweighed the potential harm.

One particularly interesting aspect of the controversy is that in the winter of 2012 scientists themselves agreed to a moratorium on *gain of function* research on H5N1—research that tries to create highly virulent forms of pathogens—until concerns and proper safeguards could be discussed. The 2012 moratorium had initially been proposed to last for sixty days, but ultimately lasted almost a year. Such self-imposed restrictions are rare, but are critical to maintaining public confidence in science. However, in October 2014 the US government issued a new moratorium banning funding of new research on gain of function, not because of fears of bioterrorism but because it was discovered that the key US government research centres had mishandled potentially dangerous samples of other pathogens.

The 'two most famous papers almost not published' found that HA, one of the two most important garments involved in flu's costume changes, determines both how transmissible *and* how virulent a particular strain of flu is likely to be. For example, some forms of HA such as those found in H1N1 can infect human cells via proteins found on the surface of cells in our noses and throats. These forms are highly transmissible, because the virus can easily find its way in and out of new hosts when it doesn't have to travel very far into our bodies. But H1N1 is not highly virulent, because the virus does not usually find suitable cells to infect deep in our lungs, and is thus less often associated with pneumonia. Other forms of HA, such as H5N1, encounter appropriate cells only deep in the lungs. They can therefore cause damage leading to pneumonia, and so are far more virulent. However, transmission of this dangerous strain is low because H5N1 particles can't infect us unless they find their way far down into our lungs.

Thanks to the now published research on ferrets, we know that only a small number of mutations are required for H5N1 to evolve the capability for airborne transmission between humans—at least for the particular strain of H5N1 virus that the researchers studied. Moreover, we are pretty sure what those mutations are. We have identified the costume change that this particular strain of virus would likely perform if it were to become pandemic—and thus we could recognize it *before* a major outbreak. If these signature mutations are found in all airborne strains, then we can detect when flu is on the path to becoming airborne (and hence likely pandemic) by tracking the genetic sequences of flu samples from domestic poultry and human patients.

Why the caveats about 'this particular virus strain'? Because influenza evolution, like any other kind of evolution, depends on where you start. While we understand the ways in which the particular strain of H5N1 that was studied by the researchers could become pandemic, we don't know if we can generalize those ideas even to other variants of H5N1, let alone to different strains such as H7N9, which is currently circulating in Asia.

Regardless of one's personal opinion about the wisdom or the utility of the 'two most famous papers almost not published', they have set important precedents for future dual-use research. The restraint that scientists showed while trying to decide whether to publish this research suggests that the research community, as well as world leaders, may at last be embracing the precautionary principle (scrutiny prior to any negative consequences, rather than after the fact). It also suggests that scientists realize that the active engagement of a broad array of stakeholders is essential to maintaining public trust in science.

Chapter 4
HIV

Our second case study is HIV, another virus likely to be familiar to most readers. HIV is the human immunodeficiency virus that causes acquired immunodeficiency syndrome, or AIDS. Once a person is infected with HIV, they may live for many years without showing any symptoms, but are still capable of transmitting the virus. After some time following the initial infection (usually several years), the virus population within the infected person begins to increase rapidly, ultimately causing immune system collapse. The HIV positive person then becomes vulnerable to opportunistic infections (see Chapter 2)—infections caused by disease agents such as the bacterium *Pneumocystis carinii*, which causes pneumonia, or the fungus *Candida albicans*; neither of these pathogens can infect a person with a normally functioning immune system. Certain types of cancer, such as Kaposi's sarcoma, also occur more frequently in people living with AIDS. Untreated, HIV infections are usually fatal within five to ten years. The proximate cause of death is usually opportunistic infection, rather than HIV per se.

HIV is a very different virus from influenza; it has a different mode of transmission between individuals, as well as a different evolutionary potential. HIV is transmitted in our most intimate moments, by exchange of bodily fluids. Many people think of HIV primarily as a sexually transmitted disease, because both semen and vaginal fluids carry enough virus to cause a new infection. However, our blood also carries HIV, which means that transmission can happen any time someone comes in contact with an infected person's blood. Medical personnel stick themselves with needles accidentally, and intravenous (IV) drug users share needles. Recipients of blood transfusions, especially haemophiliacs and others who need frequent transfusions, were often infected in the early days of the HIV epidemic (most blood supplies are now rigorously screened for HIV and many other blood-borne pathogens). Because breast milk also carries the virus, babies can contract HIV while nursing from their HIV-infected mothers.

Understanding routes of transmission is key to protecting both populations and individuals, who can modify their behaviour accordingly (safe sex, needle exchange programmes for IV drug users, eye protection and needle stick protocols for health workers, etc.). As we'll see later, being able to identify the most common routes of transmission also helps inform the use of limited resources for HIV treatment. But before we can understand treatment, we need to know more about HIV.

One of the biggest challenges of HIV is its extraordinary evolutionary potential. One might almost believe that HIV has a cloak of invisibility, rather than a series of costumes like influenza. The first few decades of research on HIV were nightmarish, because of HIV's uncanny ability to become invisible to our immune systems and to our treatments. We could not develop vaccines, because the virus changed too quickly—much more quickly than influenza, whose costume changes on the scale of years are problematic enough! That evolutionary prowess also means that HIV is incredibly variable around the world. So, in trying to create a vaccine, we would not be tracking just one moving target, but many. We feared we would never be able to develop a drug with lasting efficacy, because HIV seemed to effortlessly become invisible to our medicines as well. In order to understand HIV, then, we have to understand the details of how this pernicious disappearing act works.

Part of HIV's invisibility comes through an insidious strategy: it hides inside our own genomes. HIV is a retrovirus, which means that it has an RNA genome that is first copied into DNA by a complex viral protein, *reverse transcriptase* (RT). The resulting double-stranded DNA can then be integrated into our genomes by means of another viral protein, *integrase*. The fact that HIV can become 'us' is one of the reasons it is so difficult to cure.

However, HIV can only enter certain types of cells, an example of the compatibility filter described in Chapter 2. In order for HIV to enter a cell, the cell must have surface proteins (receptors) that fit a particular knob sticking out of HIV's envelope, *gp120* (glycoprotein—a protein with sugars attached to it—with a molecular weight of 120). Thus, blocking the gp120 compatibility filter should confer resistance to HIV. Remarkably, there is a mutation in humans that does almost exactly that. HIV actually needs to use two receptors to enter the cell: the primary receptor for gp120, which is called CD4, and a co-receptor, called CCR5. Humans with the CCR5-Δ32 mutation lack the co-receptor for gp120 and are hence resistant to HIV infection. However, to have complete protection from HIV, a person must have two copies of this mutation, one on each strand of DNA. People with a single copy of CCR5-Δ32 (heterozygotes) can still be infected and become symptomatic, though they are still more resistant than people with no copies at all.

Only three cell types have the appropriate receptors to bind with gp120, and all three are part of our immune system. It is because HIV targets immune cells that infection by HIV results in immunodeficiency. The virus hides in these cells until it is activated. Once activated, the virus begins to replicate, ultimately resulting in the death of these immune cells and weakening our ability to respond to other infections.

As noted in Chapter 3 on influenza, mutations happen at random, without respect to whether or not they are going to be advantageous to the virus. The mutation rate of a virus, then, is critical to understanding how easily (and hence how frequently) any given mutation can occur. Intuitively, we might expect HIV to have a much higher mutation rate than influenza since it evolves so quickly. And HIV's mutation rate is indeed more than ten times higher than influenza's.

Interestingly, estimates of the mutation rate for HIV depend strongly on context—for example, when we measure mutation in viruses within humans, rather than in a test tube.

HIV replication uses two distinct enzymes. One is the virus's own RT, which as described previously converts viral RNA into DNA. The DNA versions of the viral genome which have been integrated into our own DNA are copied by a second enzyme, our own RNA polymerase. These new RNA genomes are then repackaged into the virus particles that emerge from one cell to infect another. Most HIV mutations come from the reverse transcription step. The HIV RT enzyme makes more mistakes than the enzyme used by influenza, so HIV's mutation rate is higher than that of flu.

Mutation is not the only source of variation for HIV. Unlike influenza, which has a segmented genome and so can combine different viral segments from multiple viruses, HIV exchanges portions of its single-piece genome with portions of the genomes of other HIV viruses, a process called recombination. However, recombination as practised by HIV is fundamentally different from recombination in organisms such as humans, fruit flies, or pea plants. Recombination happens during the reverse transcription step, when the information in the RNA is copied into DNA. The viral RT sometimes switches from one template, the viral genome being copied, to the other (and back again). This process is called template switching. To understand template switching, imagine that you were using tracing paper to trace two parallel lines, but you are only allowed to trace one line at a time. You start at the left end of one line and move to the right. Now imagine that your tracing paper shifts up or down at random, such that sometimes you are tracing the top line and sometimes you are tracing the bottom line, but always drawing from left to right. In the end, you will have drawn a single straight line, but it will contain copies of parts of both lines. Similarly, recombinant HIV genomes contain all the parts of a single genome, but recombined from two different copies.

Because of mutation and recombination, HIV is constantly changing, to the point that it seems able to become invisible. Because vaccines rely on an immune 'photographic memory' of what a pathogen target looks like, designing a vaccine against HIV has proved extraordinarily difficult, as mentioned earlier. But HIV's invisibility is perhaps most notorious in its astonishing ability to render drugs useless, because it evolves resistance so quickly within an individual host.

We have already discussed the human mutation CCR5-Δ32, which confers resistance to HIV by blocking the compatibility filter. As it turns out, the mutation was already present in human populations before the HIV epidemic. While HIV has likely been infecting humans only for about a century, the CCR5-Δ32 mutation has been found in DNA from ancient human remains. We thus have direct evidence that the CCR5-Δ32 mutation has been around for nearly 3,000 years. Because HIV is much younger than that, and because the CCR5-Δ32 mutation is common in some human populations, researchers speculated that CCR5-Δ32 had risen to relatively high frequency because it protected against some older pathogen, such as bubonic plague or smallpox. However, careful analyses of the CCR5-Δ32 gene and its surrounding DNA revealed that the high frequencies today are most likely a happy accident—the result of genetic drift rather than natural selection. Other, less well-known genes conferring resistance to HIV also appear to be far more ancient than HIV.

In contrast to resistance mutations in the human genome, the resistance of HIV to drug therapies frequently arises from new virus mutations within individual humans, though resistant strains are sometimes transmitted from person to person. Despite these challenges, a regimen of *highly active anti-retroviral therapies (HAART)*, developed in the mid-1990s, is extraordinarily effective against HIV. HAART uses a combination of three drugs to reduce HIV proliferation. Generally, the drugs work to directly block HIV reverse transcription, in two different ways. One class of drugs acts by tricking the RT enzyme into incorporating chemicals that stop the extension of the RNA genome. These chemicals look like the building blocks used by RT, but function differently. Once one of these chemicals is incorporated, the enzyme can't continue synthesizing the genome. This class of drugs is called *nucleoside reverse transcriptase inhibitors (NRTIs)*; two different NRTIs are usually used in HAART. The other class of drugs directly binds to the RT, stopping it from working. These drugs are called *non-nucleoside reverse transcriptase inhibitors (NNRTI)*; usually only one NNRTI is used in HAART to complement the NRTIs.

The mutations that make HIV resistant to NNRTI (for example) are extremely improbable. However, even an event that is unlikely on a case-by-case basis can become common if it has sufficient opportunities to happen. Individual HIV genomes don't last long inside a human: a given HIV virion in the bloodstream survives for about six hours. Because the total number of virions is approximately constant, that must mean that virions are replaced by new ones about four times per day. In addition, each person infected with HIV has tens of millions of virions in their body. Thus there are hundreds of millions of cycles of replication, and hence opportunities for mutation, every few days. We can use a lottery analogy: if you bought hundreds of millions of lottery tickets, you would presumably eventually win the jackpot. In other words, because there are so many viruses turning over so quickly within an infected individual, even improbable mutations will happen eventually.

To understand why HAART is successful, one just needs to remember two things: first, that mutations happen at random; and second, the basic rule of probability about the co-occurrence of independent events. In order for the virus to evade HAART, it needs three independent mutations, one for each of the three drugs. Because the mutations are independent, the chance of their happening in the same individual is the product of the probability of each of them happening independently. That is, if the chance of each event were 0.5, then the chance of two such events would be 0.5×0.5, and for three, $0.5 \times 0.5 \times 0.5$. Now imagine that the probability of each individual mutation happening is much, much smaller than 0.5. Instead of 'extremely improbable', we are dealing with 'extremely improbable cubed', so that even with tens of millions of viruses and hundreds of millions of replication cycles, resistance is going to take a very long time to arise, if it ever does.

Anti-retroviral therapy was once reserved for patients with full-blown AIDS, in part because of the problems of drug resistance and limited resources. However, in 2013 an exciting new paradigm was announced by the World Health Organization: 'treatment as prevention'. Under this strategy, infected but otherwise healthy patients are given treatment to help reduce transmission. People on drug therapy have fewer circulating viruses in their bodily fluids than people who are not being treated, so people who are being treated are less likely to transmit the virus. At the level of the individual, people on treatment will remain healthier, happier, and productive for much longer. Some may never even become symptomatic.

However, HAART is a treatment, not a cure. Patients need to take the drugs every day, or the virus will start to increase again, because as mentioned earlier, there are copies of the virus hiding inside our own cells that are not affected by HAART. Indeed, interrupting therapy quickly results in virus numbers rebounding to pre-treatment levels. In order to completely cure an HIV infection, then, we would have to eradicate all the cells in our own bodies whose genomes unwittingly harbour HIV. Because the three cell types containing integrated copies of the virus are derived from bone marrow, doctors have actually tried to strategically destroy, then replace bone marrow, as is done for certain types of cancer such as leukaemia.

First, chemotherapy is used to eliminate all cells that might be infected with HIV, even though some are probably uninfected. However, this destroys key components of our immune systems, so we cannot survive for long without these cell types. So next, bone marrow from uninfected donors is transplanted into the patient, giving rise to new, uninfected immune cells. Simultaneously, aggressive antiviral therapy to destroy any viruses currently circulating in the blood is used throughout the chemotherapy and transplant process, with the goal of preventing infection of the newly produced immune cells.

In one patient, Timothy Ray Brown, the virus remains undetectable after more than four years. However, in two other patients detectable levels of HIV were present within a year following treatment. The circumstances were not identical between patients: Brown received a transplant from a donor who had two copies of CCR5-Δ32, the mutation that confers resistance to HIV by blocking the gp120 compatibility filter. The other patients received transplants from donors with only a single copy. Their new bone marrow then had only partial resistance to HIV infection.

Unfortunately, because matches between bone marrow donors and recipients are hard to get to begin with, finding a donor who is a match *and* has two copies of CCR5-Δ32 is very unlikely. For that reason alone, this treatment will never be available as a widespread cure. Moreover, the procedure requires extensive hospitalization and is thus not suitable for most of the millions of people infected with HIV. However, the significance of Timothy Ray Brown's cure is enormous, and his success will undoubtedly inspire treatments that can be used more widely. For example, the cure underscores the importance of the CCR5-Δ32 mutation, which potentially can drive new treatments based on the altered function of this gene.

One pressing question in HIV research, and in infectious disease research in general, is 'why now'? Where did HIV come from, and how did it so quickly become a worldwide threat to health and economic stability? If we can understand the answers to these questions, we may be better able to prevent or at least slow down the next emerging disease.

Researchers have used two primary tools to understand the emergence of HIV: contact networks (discussed in Chapter 3) and phylogenetic trees. A phylogenetic tree is one of the fundamental tools of evolutionary biology. It is a way of grouping organisms by similarity, which in turn (if you do it carefully) also groups them by relatedness. Figure 5 shows the phylogenetic trees for HIV and for influenza. Nowadays, most phylogenies are built using genetic information. The more recently two organisms share a common ancestor, the more closely related they are, and the more similar their genomes will be. We use phylogenetic trees to show relatedness by placing more closely related genomes closer together on a phylogeny, and placing more distantly related ones farther apart. Our ability to build phylogenetic trees relies, once again, on the random nature (and relatively constant rate) of mutation: genome similarity is assessed in terms of numbers of mutations that differ between two organisms. But we can do more with phylogenetic trees than just understand relatedness. We build phylogenetic trees because by analysing the shape of the tree, we can understand what kind of evolutionary processes have occurred, and over what time scales.

If mutations happen at similar rates in closely related species, which is almost always true, then we can estimate time simply by counting the number of mutations. If two viruses differ by seven

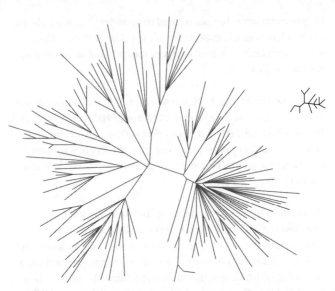

5. HIV (left, larger) is characterized by extensive genetic variation at any given time, with strains persisting for long periods of time. Influenza (right, smaller) is characterized by little variation at any given time, and strains replacing one another, rather than coexisting, over time.

mutations they are more closely related, and share a common ancestor more recently, than two viruses of the same type that vary by, say, twenty mutations. On a phylogenetic tree, the length of the branches is proportional to the number of mutations, and hence is proportional to time.

However, there's more useful information in a phylogenetic tree than just branch length: tree shape can also tell us a lot about virus evolution. Comparing a tree of influenza with a tree of HIV can give an instant intuitive understanding. The tree of influenza has a few, short branches close to the trunk. This shape reflects the fact that the majority of flu viruses do not persist in the population for long, at least not at very high frequencies. With flu, new mutants quickly take over the population, replacing old varieties. HIV trees are much more complex. It's difficult to identify a core trunk because there are so many long branches. In contrast to influenza, new mutations of HIV tend to coexist with old strains for a long time, evolving at the same time but independently.

Our best guess is that the ancestor of HIV as we know it today was contracted by some unlucky human from an infected chimpanzee butchered for food. But why did HIV become pandemic *now*? SIV, the group of viruses ancestral to HIV, has been around for thousands of years, so it seems likely that people have been exposed to them for a long time. Phylogenetic methods using both contemporary viruses and old blood samples that have been carefully stored in hospital freezers tell us that the origin of the most widespread form, the M group of HIV-1, occurred sometime between 1910 and 1930, though the original zoonotic event (the jump from chimpanzees into humans) may have occurred earlier. Other introductions of less common forms of HIV-1 occurred independently, in some cases much earlier than the M group, but these also seem to have increased in prevalence at the same time. Was something going on at that time that caused the current pandemic?

To think about this problem, we first have to understand the transfer of a pathogen from a non-human host to a human (zoonosis, see Chapter 1). Zoonoses follow two typical patterns. A zoonosis with $R_0 < 1$ in the human population, such that each human infection gives rise to less than one additional infected human, is called a spillover event. Individual infected people may be severely ill or die, but a true between-species jump or host shift won't happen because the transmission between humans is too low. On the other hand, if R_0 is even slightly greater than 1, the minimum value for persistence, then the pathogen can successfully shift hosts. Once the pathogen has started to circulate among humans, mutations may arise that help the pathogen adapt to its new host. In other words, these mutations open the compatibility filter farther and farther.

As discussed before, mutations are random; the probability of a given mutation is proportional to the number of genomes available to mutate. It is therefore critical to respond quickly to initial zoonotic events in order to limit the total mutation rate by keeping the number of human infections small. For example, in 2003 an outbreak of monkeypox virus—the first in the western hemisphere—occurred in the US as a result of a two-step host shift from a single shipment of infected Gambian pouched rats from Africa, to prairie dogs reared in captivity for the pet trade, to humans. In Africa, human-to-human transmission has evolved at least once (likely several times). However, because the patients were quickly given medical care, and because of good hygiene in the treatment facilities, human-to-human transmission did not evolve in the US and the epidemic was stopped after just seventy-one cases, with no fatalities.

The simplest argument for the current HIV pandemic, of course, is that nothing has changed—we have just been unlucky. According to this argument, the probability of SIV entering a human (passing the encounter filter) and evolving the capacity for transmission between humans (opening the compatibility filter) has been constant over time; the early 20th century just happens to be the one time it was successful. This argument is unsatisfying. Even if the probability of a successful host shift happening at any particular time is low, SIV, its primate hosts, and humans have coexisted for so long that it seems unlikely that such chimpanzee-to-human transmission has never happened before.

The most widely accepted hypothesis for HIV emergence is that successful shifts from primates to humans have indeed happened many times, but went unnoticed by the rest of the world because they failed to spread beyond the original infected community. (A similar process has happened with the Ebola virus: small outbreaks have probably been going on in isolated human populations for centuries or millennia, and have been recorded over the past forty years. It has only caught the serious attention of the West with its emergence in the urban populations of West Africa in 2014.) However, the most recent HIV shift to humans coincided with a change in human demography and sociology that facilitated transmission. This particular host shift coincided with the urbanization of Africa, which had been going on for some time, as well as the construction of roads linking many communities that had previously been isolated. Political unrest, the sexual revolution, and increased global mobility also coincided with this particular host shift.

Other researchers have argued that a simple event such as the entry of contaminated chimpanzee blood into a wound is insufficient to trigger a zoonotic shift, and that SIV got an unintentional helping hand from humans along the evolutionary road to becoming human-adapted HIV. By reusing non-sterilized syringes, medical practice may have facilitated viral persistence in humans until the mutations allowing human-to-human transmission arose.

These two hypotheses—urbanization and unsterile injections—are not mutually exclusive and may well have worked in concert to spread the virus. We will never know for certain, but by asking where HIV came from we have learned important lessons that we are already using to restrict the spread of other pathogens.

Chapter 5
Cholera

Cholera has a foundational role in any discussion of infectious disease. Cholera gave rise to Koch's postulates, one of the pillars of epidemiology. These postulates state that identifying a particular organism as the causative agent of a disease requires that (1) the organism is found in diseased people but not healthy ones, (2) the organism can be isolated from diseased people and grown in culture, (3) the laboratory-cultured organism will cause disease in a new host, and (4) the organism can be re-isolated from the newly infected host. Cholera also led to the recognition that preventive measures should focus on providing clean water, which in the process closed the encounter filter for a vast number of other water-borne pathogens.

The bacterium *Vibrio cholerae* is the cause of the diarrhoeal disease known as cholera. *V. cholerae* is a large and diverse species. New samples are assigned to types based on whether or not a particular sample reacts with antibodies produced by a mammal in response to infection by a known type. The antibodies are very specific, and only react with the type of cholera that was injected into the mammal that produced the antibodies. Thus, these antibodies can be used to identify different strains of *V. cholerae*. So, if a new sample reacts with antibodies from an animal injected with a known strain of O1, it is also an O1 type. These groups are called *serotypes*, meaning 'types based on serum', because antibodies are isolated from the blood (or serum). Two serotypes, O1 and O139, are responsible for most epidemics. Even within these serotypes, cholera bacteria can only cause epidemics if they carry at least two special genes: one to overcome the compatibility filter, and one to open the encounter filter.

To become infected with cholera, you have to ingest a huge number of the bacteria—approximately one million of them. Stomach acid, in addition to digesting our food, protects us by killing all manner of living things that we accidentally eat or drink, including cholera. Food acts to neutralize stomach acid; on a completely empty stomach, one hundred *trillion* bacteria are required to reliably produce infection in humans, 100,000 times more bacteria than when ingested with food. With that many bacteria, some can survive the gauntlet of stomach acid to make it through to the small intestine.

Bacteria that survive the stomach acid must also be able to infect cells in the small intestine. At a minimum, cholera must possess a cluster of genes involved in creating the toxin co-regulated pilus, or TCP. TCP is an essential component of the compatibility factor—without it, no illness occurs. Many other genes enhance colonization abilities, but TCP is the only one that is absolutely essential. Remarkably, even after colonization illness usually does not result unless the gene for cholera enterotoxin (CT) is expressed; that is, cholera is infectious but not virulent. Virulence and transmission are strongly correlated in cholera; CT is essential for between-host transmission of cholera (its exit strategy). CT disrupts water regulation in the intestine, producing a flood of diarrhoea that leads to dehydration and death for the host but also pushes cholera back out into the environment, allowing it to encounter new hosts.

The bright spot in all of these horrific symptoms is that treatment for cholera is remarkably straightforward. Just giving cholera victims a simple oral rehydration solution containing sugar and salt can drastically reduce death rates, or even prevent death altogether. Antibiotics are useful, but as a secondary defence. The most important benefit of antibiotics is that they shorten the infectious period, and thus can reduce the risk of transmission.

Cholera has played an important role in the history of epidemiology. Snow's discovery that cholera was spread by a contagious agent, and localizing that agent to a particular water pump during a cholera outbreak in mid-19th-century London, is arguably the first case of epidemiology as systematic detective work.

Snow's insights continue to be useful today: closing the encounter filter by setting up water purification and water treatment plants is an excellent way to prevent cholera epidemics. However, water purification by boiling (a low-tech solution that can be implemented in remote or less developed areas) requires enormous amounts of firewood, which can be dangerous to retrieve in politically unstable areas, and can lead to deforestation. Higher-tech solutions such as treatment plants or water purification via chemicals are expensive and can be logistically difficult. A recent innovation in low-tech, effective intervention is to filter water through four thicknesses of sari cloth, which can reduce infection rates by 50 per cent.

However, even with water treatment systems in place, infected people can spread cholera within their own households. Analysing the social network of cholera epidemics shows that infections spread much more rapidly within households than between them, likely due to contamination of water or food by cholera carried on the hands of caretakers. Accordingly, public health agencies have promoted water storage vessels with narrow mouths and spigots (rather than traditional open-mouthed buckets) so that infected people cannot contaminate the household's supply by dipping their hands or clothes in the water. Such interventions have reduced cholera transmission rates by almost 40 per cent.

How does cholera evolve? In the Red Queen race against hosts, bacteria generally use complete costume changes less often than viruses do. Because the biochemical machinery of bacteria differs significantly from ours, we can fight back by trying to poison the bacteria with antibacterial compounds borrowed from other organisms such as fungi (Chapter 1). This strategy usually fails on viruses, because they use so many of our own biochemical pathways that we would be poisoning ourselves at the same time. Another reason for the difference is that because bacteria mutate many times slower than viruses, they can't accumulate individual changes fast enough to hide effectively from our immune systems. Instead of evasion, they focus on resistance to host countermeasures.

Rather than switching their entire wardrobe, bacteria such as *V. cholerae* accessorize by gaining (and losing) accessories (countermeasures) according to the demands natural selection makes of them at any given time. If natural selection demands a feather boa, and one is available in the costume box (i.e. the local environment), any bacterium that picks it up will prosper. That is, the bacterium with the boa will have more descendants than the ones without it—natural selection in the usual sense. However, to a bacterium even a feather boa is heavy, so if it is not explicitly required for survival it is in the bacterium's best interest to drop it.

Obviously bacteria don't wear boas. Instead, they gain and lose genes. One way to do this is by acquiring mobile genetic elements from other bacteria. Another source of useful novel genes is from viruses that infect the bacteria. Both these mechanisms are referred to as lateral gene transfer (LGT for short), because they involve the movement of genes among organisms within generations (laterally), rather than between generations (vertically). Bacteria reproduce by dividing rather than having offspring as animals do, but the creation of new individuals isn't required for LGT, just contact between existing organisms.

Cholera

One of our favourite examples of evolution in real time is antibiotic resistance in bacteria, which is usually accomplished by LGT, often via genes carried on plasmids (small circular pieces of DNA that are separate from the chromosome). Cholera is no exception. While antibiotics are not required to cure cholera, they do shorten the duration of the infectious period, and the symptoms. Heavy use of antibiotics creates a scenario where resistance will be selected, if it is present.

Unlike in viruses, drug resistance in bacteria does not generally arise as a result of new mutations, for several reasons. First, as already mentioned, bacterial mutation rates are usually much lower than viral rates—this reduces bacteria's ability to evolve new drug resistance mechanisms. Second, bacteria are more likely to trade genes among themselves—that is, participate in LGT—than viruses are. Two of the most infamous cases of drug resistance in bacteria, methicillin-resistant *Staphylococcus aureus* (MRSA) and a new scourge, carbapenem-resistant enterobacteriaceae (CRE), are caused by genes for resistance to different antibiotics.

Cholera acquires resistance primarily by gaining a piece of DNA called SXT, which is similar to a plasmid but is linear rather than circular. Once it gains antibiotic resistance, a bacterium will be more successful than one without it as long as antibiotics are in use. When antibiotic use ceases, however, resistance can be lost. Bacteria with big genomes take longer to replicate than bacteria with small ones, so bacteria containing lots of integrated antibiotic resistance genes will take longer in the absence of antibiotic to replicate than bacteria without such genes. This can be a significant handicap in a rapidly growing population, and is referred to as the *cost of resistance*.

Just as DNA can be integrated into the genome, it can also pop out again. If that happens, the bacterium with the smaller genome may have an advantage. Alternatively, if the antibiotic resistance genes are on plasmids, rather than in the chromosome itself, the plasmids themselves may be lost at random through genetic drift if they do not give the bacteria any advantage. In other bacterial systems, the cost of resistance may be driven by the metabolic costs of the resistance gene, which may make the organism expend a lot of energy pumping toxins out of its cells, or because the organism switches to a biochemical pathway that is immune to the effects of the antibiotic but less efficient at its metabolic role.

Even as cholera bacteria parasitize us, they too can be parasitized—by viruses. Remarkably, as previously mentioned, bacteria can acquire useful genes from their viral parasites—although perhaps this isn't all that remarkable when we think about it. Natural selection rewards organisms for being opportunistic, so in some circumstances a virus that gives something useful to its host is more likely to persist than one that doesn't. To understand what kind of circumstance will allow cholera to pick up genetic novelties from its viruses, we have to know a little bit more about the viruses that infect bacteria: the *phages*.

One common type of phage is the temperate phage, which can follow two strategies. The first is lysogeny: once a phage enters the cell, its DNA is incorporated into the genome of the bacterium. The phage's DNA is now called a *prophage*. The prophage is replicated along with the bacterium's own DNA, spreading to all the offspring of the original infected organism. It's a peaceable kingdom—unless the phage gets a biochemical signal that tells it that it is threatened. In that case, the phage may exit non-destructively, or it may adopt a lytic strategy.

In the lytic strategy, the phage turns its bacterial host into a virus production factory, ultimately killing the bacterium by bursting ('lysing') the cell once enough offspring are created. These new phage can go on to infect other bacteria, and pursue either the lysogenic or lytic strategy depending on environmental conditions.

As mentioned earlier, only a few strains of *V. cholerae* carry the toxin gene CT. CT is a gift carried by the temperate phage CTXɸ to its host. Once CTXɸ is ensconced in the cholera genome, the toxin can be expressed and increase transmission (and hence R_0). But phages, even temperate phages, are not altruistic. CT increases the fitness of the bacteria, but it also increases the fitness of the (now) prophage, which multiplies right along with the bacteria inside the patient's gut.

The other essential genetic ingredient for pandemic cholera is TCP, which as discussed earlier enables cholera to colonize the small intestine. TCP has another function as well: it is the receptor for the phage CTXɸ. Receptors are part of the host compatibility filter for viruses. Without the correct match between virus and receptor, infection can't occur. By expressing TCP, cholera invites infection by CTXɸ, and thereby receives the gift of CT. It's a beautiful, if sinister, example of coevolution: the two components that are necessary for high transmission of cholera (and therefore also of the prophage) are part of an interdependent system assuring the fitness of both parties.

But this pretty scenario of invitations and gifts is a profound misreading of what is more accurately viewed as an ongoing feud. The bacteria do not want the phages to come to the party, gift or no; even if the phage doesn't kill when it exits, it is still exerting a cost, however small, on the bacterium. Instead, the phage is a party crasher. It uses TCP as a receptor because TCP is something the bacterium needs for its own sake. And CT is not a gift. The phage carry it only because it increases its own fitness. If its fitness can increase along with the bacterium's, fine, but the only reason it works that way is because the phage is integrated into the bacterial genome, and so their fitness is inextricably linked. But if a mutation or new chunk of DNA were to appear that increased viral fitness still further at the expense of the bacterium, or that allowed the bacterium to maintain CT while getting rid of the rest of the party-crashing prophage, natural selection would optimize such changes and all illusions of polite society would vanish.

In fact, there is evidence for the darker version of this story. Digging a little deeper, researchers have learned that the genes coding for CT are probably a recent acquisition by the phage. There are numerous related phages that do not carry CT, but still use TCP as their receptor. Moreover, the composition of the CT genes suggests that the CT genes are newer than the rest of the genome. Not only bacteria, but also the viruses that parasitize them, can accessorize for their own benefit.

Why hasn't TCP evolved so that the CTX phage can't use it, particularly since many of these phages don't even bring CT with them? Phage infection probably doesn't hurt the cholera bacteria very much—even when threatened, this phage exits the cell without killing it. So there's little selective pressure for the bacteria to resist infection by altering TCP, especially given that they need TCP for intestinal colonization.

Other phages that infect cholera behave more like traditional predators which always kill their prey. These phages are *obligately* lytic; they can only survive by lysing or bursting their host. In other words, if they infect a bacterium, it's doomed. The best known of these lytic phages are known as the JSF phage group; they use a different receptor from CTXφ to gain entry to the cholera bacteria.

In regions where cholera is endemic, epidemics occur seasonally. Scientists have recently noticed that epidemics in the Ganges River Delta tend to start when there are lower numbers of lytic phages in the water and stop when there are more lytic phages. Moreover, the relative abundance of phage in patients with cholera reflects their relative abundance in the aquatic environment: fewer lytic phages in patients early in the epidemic, more later in the epidemic. These observations suggest that lytic phage epidemics among cholera might ride along on top of the cholera epidemic occurring in humans, possibly even helping to control the epidemic.

Phages could be used to control cholera in individuals as well as at the population level. This form of treatment—phage therapy—has been around at least since the 1920s, when it was developed as a treatment for dysentery, a diarrhoeal disease like cholera that is caused by a different bacterium. The big advantage of phage therapy is that many phages are specific to a particular bacterium: there are no side effects. Conventional antibiotics attack not only unfriendly bacteria but also the essential bacteria in our bodies; many women have had the experience of suffering from yeast infections when antibiotics have knocked out the bacteria that normally inhabit their reproductive tracts. Successful, well-designed phage therapy would kill the bad bacteria while leaving the good guys alone.

The downside of phage therapy is that it tries to harness a living system that is capable of evolution. Once phages are introduced to a patient, they can evolve in any way natural selection directs them, including in ways that could make people sicker, as in the case of CT. One possible safeguard that could reduce such risks of phage therapy is to limit therapeutic phages' capability to exchange genes with the bacteria they infect. Phage evolvability may be one reason that phage therapy has not been embraced outside of Russia and Georgia, though very few adverse incidents involving phage therapy have been reported in the last sixty years. Phage therapy is enjoying a resurgence of interest around the world, in part due to the rise in antibiotic resistance, but also in part due to the apparently beneficial effects of lytic phages at the population level.

The seasonality of cholera epidemics is worth a closer look. In Bangladesh, phages parasitizing cholera fluctuate seasonally as well. These fluctuations seem to track the density of cholera in a pattern that is well known to ecologists as the pattern of regular (animal–animal or animal–plant) predator–prey systems: the prey (cholera) increase first, then predators (phage) increase, causing prey to decrease once again. Once prey decrease, the predator of course decreases as well, having nothing to eat, allowing prey to increase once again and creating cycles of abundance. Thus, rather than the phage controlling the abundance of their prey, *V. cholerae*, the prey might well drive the abundance of the predator. Support for this idea comes from the observation that cholera epidemics in Haiti also show seasonality, but there doesn't seem to be any phage in the environment. Thus, either seasonality is driven by different mechanisms in the two locations, or the phage seasonality is a consequence rather than a cause of bacterial seasonality.

Contrary to what one might expect of an organism transmitted through drinking water, cholera thrives in salt water. It can also persist in fresh water, if the water is warm enough and contains enough nutrients. Epidemics in Bangladesh closely track surface sea water temperatures, for two reasons. First, warm sea surface water temperatures are associated with severe storms, which in turn cause flooding. Flooding worsens existing sanitation problems, co-mingling drinking water and sewage, and facilitating transmission of cholera.

Second, warm sea surface temperatures (particularly in association with large amounts of nutrients) cause blooms of tiny plants called phytoplankton. The phytoplankton are food for zooplankton—tiny floating marine animals. Cholera can stick to the exoskeletons of shrimp-like zooplankton known as copepods, whose bodies are made of a substance called chitin. Remember that a person needs to swallow huge numbers of cholera bacteria in order for any of them to survive our stomach acid. An individual copepod can accumulate ten thousand cholera bacteria: swallowing such a copepod is like ingesting a cholera bomb. If one such copepod arrives on a stomach full of food, enough cholera can easily be delivered to cause disease, while swallowing water with just a few free-living bacteria is unlikely to harm anyone. The ability of large numbers of cholera to stick to copepods has been used to explain how cholera outbreaks could arise from environmental sources of cholera, rather than from infected patients.

As with most other areas of science that matter at all, some parts of the cholera story are well accepted by the scientific community, while other parts are not. For example, scientists have long been puzzled by the fact that cholera behaves differently depending on the conditions under which it was reared. Cholera reared in laboratory culture is the standard on which estimates of the infectious dose (the number of particles required to make a person ill) are generally calculated. However, as lab-reared cholera fed to a volunteer go through the process of infecting the gut and being expelled in diarrhoea, these same bacteria can change to a *hyperinfectious* state. Far fewer numbers of these hyperinfectious bacteria are required to infect a new host. Without invoking such a hyperinfectious state, it's hard to explain how cholera can spread through a population so incredibly quickly—for example, there were 30,000 cases in just the first week of the 1991 cholera epidemic in Peru.

If hyperinfectious cholera reaches another human gut, it remains in the hyperinfectious state (as long as it doesn't get killed by lytic phage or hit with antibiotics). On the other hand, if it leaves a patient's bowels, enters the water, and fails to get taken up by another human victim for five to twenty-four hours, it undergoes another fundamental physiological change to a very different state called either 'viable but non-culturable' or 'active but non-culturable'. You can already see the controversy: even though this phenomenon has been known for more than thirty years, we can't even agree on what to call it! The non-culturable form of cholera has gained attention as a potential environmental reservoir for new cholera outbreaks. However, it's unknown whether or not this process is reversible, in particular, whether or not the bacteria can recover their ability to colonize humans after entering the non-culturable state.

An alternative environmental reservoir for cholera could come from the *persister* phenotype assumed by some cells after they enter water. When *V. cholerae* is starved for nutrients, as happens when it leaves the human gut and enters a water supply, some cells can enter this persistent state. Like the non-culturable states, the persistent state seems to involve dormancy, and involves changes in gene expression and morphology. However, persister bacteria *can* be cultured, and have been demonstrated experimentally to reawaken when provided with sufficient resources, particularly chitin.

One example of the importance of understanding sources of cholera outbreaks and the virulence of genes themselves comes from the ongoing cholera epidemic in Haiti. The tragedy of the 2010 earthquake in Haiti was heightened by an outbreak of cholera, with over 470,000 cases reported and 6,631 people dead in the first year. Haiti had been free of cholera cases for at least one hundred years, which raised the immediate question of how the disease had arrived. Analyses ranging from serotyping, to simple comparison of presence and absence of particular genes, to sophisticated phylogenetic analyses, have all suggested that the strains did not come from a local environmental source, such as the Gulf of Mexico.

Instead, the strains isolated from Haitian patients were most similar to strains from South East Asia, suggesting that they may have arrived with people from this area, or people who recently visited there—in this case, UN peacekeepers from Nepal. In addition, the camp of the peacekeepers was located on a tributary of the Artibonite River, which was identified as the source of the Haitian outbreak, although cholera rapidly spread throughout the country.

Chapter 6
Malaria

Malaria might be the most important infectious disease on the planet. Compared to the infectious diseases discussed in the previous chapters, it is less frightening to people in temperate, developed countries—not because it is less infectious or less virulent, but because in modern times it rarely reaches out of the tropics, being limited by the ecological niche of its mosquito vectors. Unlike cholera, malaria tends to be *endemic*—maintaining a relatively constant level in the population over time—rather than occurring in intense epidemic outbreaks. Typical of endemic disease, the most widespread strains of malaria are typically chronic and debilitating, rather than causing acute infection and death. The exception is falciparum malaria, most common in tropical sub-Saharan Africa. The malnutrition and anaemia associated with chronic malaria are associated with poorer educational outcomes in children, while acute malaria can lead to chronic neurological problems. Combining these non-lethal effects common to all malaria species with the lethal effects of falciparum, the cumulative impact of malaria on humanity is enormous.

Public health officials measure the impact of chronic diseases in terms of *disability-adjusted life years* (DALYs), which take into account both the loss of life and the loss of productivity and happiness due to a disease. Coming up with appropriate weights poses obvious ethical challenges. Is one year of life with a chronic, crippling disease equivalent to six months of healthy life? Three months? One month? How should one compare the impact of death or disability in an infant, a middle-aged person, or an elderly person? Nevertheless, DALY calculations account for the fact that the chronic effects of disease on people living with disease can be just as important, if not more important, than disease-induced deaths. In 2010, malaria accounted for more lost DALYs than any other infectious disease, narrowly edging out HIV/AIDS. Although hard evidence is difficult to come by—poor countries tend to be malarial while rich ones do not—researchers have suggested that eliminating malaria could increase economic growth rates by several percentage points, the difference between a struggling economy and a healthy one.

Although every infectious disease has its bizarre and intriguing quirks, malaria is more complex than the other diseases we have discussed so far. It is caused by a protozoan, a single-celled organism whose genetic material (unlike in bacteria) is confined within a nucleus. Its genome comprises about twenty-three million base pairs of DNA, thousands of times larger than the viral genomes of HIV and influenza and about five times larger than cholera's genome.

Malaria's complexity also stems from its *vector-borne* nature; it is transmitted from one human to another via various species of *Anopheles* mosquitoes. Cholera adjusts its biochemistry to function alternately as a free-living organism in the ocean and as a pathogen in the human gut. Malaria has an even more challenging problem; it adjusts its biochemistry to two different biological environments (the human host and mosquito vector), and to multiple organs within each host (human blood and liver; mosquito gut and salivary glands). Biological environments represent bigger challenges for parasitic organisms than physical environments. Desiccation and ultraviolet light are dangerous threats to parasites travelling through the physical environment outside the host, but they are passive. In contrast, host organisms take active steps to destroy parasitic hitchhikers by attacking them with immune defences.

Four species of malaria commonly infect humans. In order of decreasing severity, the malaria species are *Plasmodium falciparum*, *P. vivax*, *P. ovale*, and *P. malariae*. (Malaria species are referred to by the genus name *Plasmodium*, which can be abbreviated as *P.*, and their species name.) A fifth species, *P. knowlesi*, known originally as a disease of macaques, is emerging as a disease of humans in South East Asia, but so far only monkey-to-human (via mosquito) transmission, not human-to-human transmission, has been observed.

All malaria species have essentially the same life cycle. It starts with sexual reproduction (fusion of female and male *gametocytes*, the equivalent of eggs and sperm coming together) in the gut of a mosquito host, after which the next life stage (*sporozoites*) migrate to the mosquito salivary glands and are injected into the human host when the mosquito bites to get protein to feed her eggs. (Only mature female mosquitoes bite humans, which has important implications for malaria control.) The injected sporozoites migrate to the human's liver where they reproduce by simple division, migrate back to the bloodstream, and continue to multiply, infecting and destroying red blood cells as the population grows. Eventually the blood stages develop into female and male gametocytes and wait for another female mosquito to arrive and suck them up.

Malaria causes anaemia by destroying red blood cells. However, the worst symptoms occur when malaria parasites (most often *P. falciparum*) get into the brain, causing cerebral malaria. In cerebral malaria, parasites block blood flow and trigger inflammation, killing untreated patients and often causing brain damage even in patients who are treated and recover.

Malaria's most obvious symptom is fever, although fever does not itself seem to be harmful. Malarial fever recurs with characteristic frequency as new waves of parasites emerge from the liver into the blood: historically malaria strains were classified according to whether fever recurred every other day (*tertian*: *P. vivax* and *P. ovale*) or every three days (*quartan*: *P. malariae* and *P. falciparum*). In many malarial regions, patients who come to the hospital with fever and headache are automatically treated for malaria since testing is expensive and requires expertise.

Malaria's inability to move directly from one human to another opens up a wide range of possibilities for control. As Chapter 2 describes, Ronald Ross, one of the founders of disease modelling, figured out two important facts about malaria. First, he discovered that mosquitoes transmit malaria, which made it possible for the first time to prevent malaria by controlling mosquitoes, or by preventing them from biting humans (closing the encounter filter). Second, his models showed that public health agencies didn't need to completely eradicate mosquitoes to eradicate malaria—they just needed to reduce the number of mosquito bites by killing or repelling mosquitoes, until, on average, each malaria-infected person is bitten by so few mosquitoes that they lead to fewer than one new infection. The encounter filter doesn't need to be completely shut—just closed tightly enough that only a few mosquitoes can sneak through.

If you can't close the encounter filter by killing, blocking, or repelling mosquitoes in any of their life stages, you can try to close the compatibility filter. In prehistoric times, humans evolved many genetic mechanisms for closing the compatibility filter, although usually at a cost. Even before humans knew the cause of malaria, we developed drugs to block the compatibility filter by poisoning malaria within our bodies in ways that are somewhat less toxic to humans than to malaria. For example, gin and tonic was the favoured drink of British colonists in the tropics from the early 1800s on, due to the antimalarial action of the quinine found in tonic water. Most recently, we have tried to come up with vaccines to bolster our natural immunity, although so far without complete success. In what follows we will discuss all three of these compatibility-blocking strategies.

Biologists have retrieved ancient DNA from 4,000-year-old Egyptian mummies, but we know malaria is far older. Early relatives of malaria have been found in the guts of midges (biting flies) in amber, which were probably biting cold-blooded reptiles, from one hundred million years ago. However, such fossils are extremely rare, and in order to resolve the gap between one hundred million and 3,000 years ago we have to turn to the genome of malaria, and of its hosts.

Malaria parasites are part of a large, complex family, the apicomplexans, that frequently jump between hosts. Although the malaria parasites of lizards, birds, and mammals are all called *Plasmodium*, they are most likely two separate families (one that infects lizards and birds and one that infects mammals) that are more closely related to other parasites than to each other; mammalian malaria split off from the rest of the family around thirteen million years ago. The malaria species that infect humans are a similarly mixed group; they are all more closely related to various malaria parasites of non-human hosts than to each other, having split off somewhere around two to seven million years ago.

Exactly which non-human host various human malaria species jumped from, and when, is a rapidly developing and controversial story. Analyses of the genome of *P. falciparum*, the most dangerous species of human malaria, suggest that its population expanded greatly about 10,000 years ago, simultaneously with the development of agriculture and a concomitant increase in human population density. Where falciparum came from in the first place is a tougher question. While it is closely related to the chimpanzee malaria *P. reichenowi*, leading older textbooks to state that it jumped from chimpanzees into humans, two recent studies have made novel and contradictory claims. The first found more closely related malaria strains in blood samples from captive bonobos (a close relative of chimpanzees and humans); the second found more closely related strains in wild gorilla faeces. These results are still controversial; the authors of the gorilla study point out that falciparum-related infections are rare in wild chimpanzees and bonobos, and that therefore the bonobo infections are most likely to originate from humans. Regardless of our conclusions about falciparum's true origins, this tells us how tiny a window we still have into the complex ecosystem of malaria, its hosts, and their vectors.

The human genome sheds more light on the history of human–malaria interactions. Humans are not passive nurseries for malaria parasites; our immune systems are constantly evolving new ways to counter the parasite's debilitating effects. Humans have a variety of genetic anti-malaria strategies, with varying efficacy and severity of side effects. The best-known of these strategies is the sickle-cell trait, which appears in biology textbooks as an example of heterozygote advantage: individuals with one copy of the sickle-cell allele and one normal haemoglobin allele are partially tolerant of falciparum malaria, but having two copies of the allele causes crippling anaemia.

Thalassemia is another mutation similar to sickle-cell, relatively common in Mediterranean populations, that modifies red blood cells to reduce the severity of malarial symptoms at the price of anaemia. Glucose-6-phosphate-dehydrogenase (G6PD) deficiency, also common in Mediterranean populations, protects against falciparum and vivax malaria. G6PD also causes anaemia, but only under particular circumstances such as eating fava beans or taking common antimalarial drugs such as chloroquine or primaquine. Duffy negativity—the absence of the 'Duffy antigen', a protein that *P. vivax* and *P. knowlesi* target to enter red blood cells—prevents against malaria symptoms at the cost of a wide range of side effects.

Genetic analysis can estimate how long ago mutations arose. The well-known human blood type O appears to provide some protection from malaria, but it is so old—it has been around for millions of years, longer than human malaria itself—that it must originally have evolved for some reason other than malaria protection, probably to protect against some other now-unknown blood pathogen. Some variants of Duffy negativity are around 30,000 years old. G6PD deficiency arose 5,000 to 10,000 years ago, reinforcing the evidence from the falciparum genome that the risk to humans from falciparum malaria exploded around the time that agriculture developed. In contrast some sickle-cell variants are evolutionarily young—only a few hundreds or thousands of years old—reminding us that the human and malaria genomes are constantly (co)evolving.

Because these genetic protective mechanisms come with severe side effects, natural selection increases their frequencies only in regions where the risk of malaria outweighs the side effects. Elsewhere, it reduces their frequencies. Since malaria is so widespread and can have such deadly effects, it may be one of the strongest selective forces shaping the human genome in the past few thousand years. The geographic distributions of particular malaria-related genes (the Duffy antigen and sickle-cell in sub-Saharan Africa, thalassemia and G6PD deficiency around the Mediterranean) give evidence about the historical distribution of malaria. Because the side effects of malaria-protective genes are only one of the vast number of factors affecting human fitness, however, the stories told by human genetics and pathogen genes are sometimes complex. For example, researchers have traditionally assumed that the absence of the Duffy antigen in sub-Saharan Africa indicates that *P. vivax* originated there. Studies of the *P. vivax* genome complicated the story by linking vivax most closely to macaque (monkey) malarias from South East Asia, suggesting that Duffy negativity might have arisen for protection against other species of malaria or other malaria-like parasites, or after vivax made its way from Asia into Africa. Most recently, however, malaria DNA found in samples of wild gorilla faeces has again shifted the evidence back in favour of an African origin for vivax.

In addition to humans' evolved constitutive defences against malaria (systems that are in place whether or not a person has ever been infected), humans' adaptive immune systems can also help. Unfortunately, unlike the immune response to simple, acute viral diseases like measles, where immunity develops quickly and is essentially lifelong, malaria immunity develops slowly. No one completely understands why, although the huge variation in molecular markers among strains of malaria, and the ability of a single clone of malaria to switch its molecular appearance, is thought to be responsible. In high-malaria areas, people typically become tolerant to malaria as children, after they have already been infected several times. Malaria immunity generally wears off quickly, perhaps in part through the malaria parasite's interference with the human immune system.

Another problem is that humans' adaptive immunity to malaria provides more tolerance (also called *clinical immunity*) than resistance. In other words, immunity does reduce the number of parasites in the bloodstream, but its main effect is to reduce the severity of symptoms. This tolerance has two important implications: (1) people in high-malaria zones with clinical immunity won't feel sick, so they won't get treated even when treatments are available—this makes it harder to reduce malaria rates from high levels; (2) it will be correspondingly easier to keep malaria rates in check once malaria rates, and levels of clinical immunity, have been reduced.

For most of history, most humans have dealt with malaria by avoiding malarial zones (if they had a choice) or by living with it, hoping for some degree of attenuation of the symptoms through natural immunity. Our historical knowledge of malaria begins with humans' first attempts to consciously defend themselves against malaria. Humans discovered compatibility-blocking chemical defences against malaria long before they discovered the microorganisms that cause it. Jesuit priests brought the traditional medication quinine, derived from tree bark, to Europe in the early 17th century. Because South American natives chewed on the bark of the cinchona tree to stop shivering, the Jesuits guessed it might work on malarial fevers, which are often accompanied by shivering. The Jesuits got lucky; quinine doesn't actually reduce fever, but it does cure malaria by leading to the build up of toxic chemicals within blood-inhabiting stages of the malaria parasite.

While quinine can cure malaria, it is too expensive and too toxic to give it to everyone in the population regardless of whether they have malaria or not. Whenever possible, it's cheaper and safer to prevent disease by closing the encounter filter to block transmission rather than trying to close the compatibility filter once transmission has already happened. This idea applies to many diseases. Low-tech solutions like monogamy, or condoms, or clean needles, or hand sanitizer, or special water containers, work better (if you can get people to use them) than the best vaccines and treatments.

For malaria, the conclusion from this line of reasoning is that controlling malaria transmission (e.g. by covering water containers to remove suitable habitat for larval mosquitoes) may work better than treating people who are already infected. Sometimes mosquito reduction, and thus malaria control, occurs naturally as a side effect of changes in land use; changes in agricultural practice that reduced the amount of standing water available for mosquito breeding are thought to have led to declines in malaria in the northern US in the late 19th century. Of course, land use change can work in either direction. Abandonment of agricultural land in the southern US in the 1930s *increased* malaria infection. More recently, malaria in western Kenya has increased along with an increase in the number of active brick-making pits, which hold water but tend to have few mosquito-eating predators, providing a perfect habitat for larvae.

Prior to the discovery of DDT, public health authorities sometimes teamed up with engineers to reduce larval mosquito habitat by managing water—draining swamps or increasing water flow or changing water levels to make the habitat inhospitable to whatever local species of mosquito was transmitting malaria. They also sprayed oil or arsenic-based insecticides in the water to kill larvae. In a form of biological control, health authorities introduced larvae-eating fish, especially the genus *Gambusia*, which is called the mosquitofish due to its dietary habits. In the first half of the 20th century, mosquitofish were brought from North America to malarial regions all over the world, from South America to central Asia to Italy to Palestine. However, it's hard to know exactly how well they worked since they were usually combined with other control measures such as water management and chemical spraying.

While such forms of source reduction were somewhat effective in developed countries, temperate or semi-arid regions, and other areas where malaria spread slowly, they were often impractical for poor, humid, tropical countries where malaria was rampant. Paul Hermann Müller's discovery of the insecticidal properties of DDT in 1939, for which he won the Nobel Prize in 1948, revolutionized malaria control. It triggered a shift from environmental and ecological engineering focused on destroying mosquitoes in their larval habitats, to protection by killing adult mosquitoes in the vicinity of humans. Indoor residual spraying programmes apply long-lasting insecticide to surfaces in houses where mosquitoes like to land. They work extremely well if a cheap, long-lasting, relatively non-toxic (to humans) insecticide such as DDT is available. Houses may only need to be sprayed a few times a year, depending on the climate and the characteristics of the wall surfaces. In general, residual spraying works better than trying to exclude mosquitoes from houses—not only is it usually cheaper, but it kills mosquitoes rather than just excluding them, thus potentially providing some protection in the area around houses. Residual spraying programmes recorded initial successes all over the world: malaria was finally eliminated from the US in the early 1950s after decades of source reduction, while residual spraying (with DDT and with other insecticides) in many African countries significantly lowered the malaria burden, at least initially.

The second great post-war advance in malaria control was the development of chloroquine, a cheaper and relatively non-toxic biochemical variant of quinine. Chloroquine was first synthesized by German scientists after World War I. At that time the Allies controlled Java, which had most of the world's supply of quinine, depriving German troops in East Africa of this vital drug. During World War II, the tables turned when the Japanese took over Java; US researchers then developed chloroquine into an effective antimalarial, although again too late to help their soldiers (who were located this time in Sicily and South East Asia). The mass administration of chloroquine both improved individual health by curing sick people of malaria, and reduced the threat of malaria at the population level by reducing the chances that a malarial person would pass the pathogen on to a mosquito. In addition to its other advantages, chloroquine helps control the sexual stages of most malaria species, thus blocking transmission as well as helping the infected person.

The combined power of DDT and chloroquine, along with other synthetic insecticides and treatments, made global health agencies very optimistic in the 1950s that malaria could be controlled and even eradicated. However, malaria control efforts in the most resistant zones—rural districts of poor, tropical countries—ran into unanticipated problems after a few decades. Even though DDT and chloroquine were relatively cheap, non-toxic, and effective, the financial and logistical difficulties of mounting a global malaria campaign were greater than anyone had imagined.

First, like all campaigns to help people in less developed countries, malaria control programmes run into logistical, administrative, and cultural roadblocks. Does the local government actually send the supplies out to the places they're most needed? Do people steal them for other uses? Are the roads good enough to get them there? If they get there, can you train people to use them properly? Local residents may not want to use DDT, because it smells bad and stains their walls. They may resent foreign intrusion. Conflicts may break out and interrupt the programme, sending you back to square one. Funding agencies may tire of donating money after a few years, or they may decide that some other problem—feeding people, or providing them with clean water, or preventing a different disease such as Ebola—is more important.

The Global Malaria Eradication Program, which began in 1955 and aimed to eradicate malaria by 1963, encountered all of these problems, and more, before it was finally abandoned in 1969, although it did reduce the malaria mortality rate more than tenfold from its 1900 baseline. Another unforeseen problem with the campaign was the linkage of DDT use to bird deaths in North America publicized in Rachel Carson's *Silent Spring* (1962), leading to a ban on the pesticide within the US and later Canada.

Second, like all infectious disease control efforts, the enemies you're fighting are biological organisms, and they will evolve countermeasures against your control strategies. Resistance evolves both in malaria vectors (against DDT and other synthetic insecticides) and in the pathogen itself (against chloroquine and other synthetic antimalarial drugs). The basic principle of chemical control is to poison the target organism—introduce a chemical that disrupts some aspect of its physiology or biochemistry, without being too toxic to the host (for chemotherapeutic agents) or other species in the environment (for vector control agents). The target is then under very strong selection pressure to either (1) change its biology in a way that neutralizes the effects of the chemical, or (2) develop ways to detoxify the chemical or remove it from its cells.

Mosquitoes gain resistance to chloroquine by inheriting mutations that pump the chemical out of their cells. No one knows exactly when these mutations first occurred, but they spread very rapidly; chloroquine resistance in *P. falciparum* was first detected in the late 1950s in South America and South East Asia, and appeared in Africa in the 1970s. By the mid-2000s, chloroquine resistance had spread globally. Luckily, a new antimalarial drug called artemisinin, rediscovered by Chinese researchers screening historically known cures for fever, was available at that time. Artemisinin is now the first-line drug of choice for malaria treatment; however, it, too, has already seen the evolution of partial resistance so far contained to South East Asia. The World Health Organization is actively trying to prevent resistance from spreading, primarily by making sure that artemisinin is always used in combination with other antimalarial drugs to radically decrease the probability that strains of malaria will be able to evolve to resist both drugs simultaneously, much in the same way that resistance to HAART treatment for HIV is extremely rare because three drugs are used.

DDT-resistant mosquitoes have genetic modifications that either change the biochemistry of their neurons (the target of DDT), or allow them to detoxify DDT within their bodies. DDT resistance had already begun to be detected by the mid-1950s, and is widespread today, although levels of resistance vary enormously from country to country and from one mosquito species to another. Some researchers argue that DDT resistance comes in large part from heavy agricultural use (against insects other than mosquitoes, but exposing mosquitoes as a by-product), and that DDT could have been much more effective if had been restricted to use in disease control programmes. While in principle mosquito populations could also lose DDT resistance if managers stopped using DDT in an area, experiments in flies have shown that DDT resistance seems to carry little if any fitness cost, so that DDT resistance is likely to persist for a long time. Malaria control programmes now try to manage resistance by switching among a variety of different synthetic insecticides that vary in their cost, effectiveness against mosquitoes, and toxicity to humans or other insects or wildlife.

In the last few decades international efforts towards malaria eradication and control have ramped up again. Planners have learned lessons from the failures of earlier programmes: in particular, they are more aware of the importance of political and cultural context, of using different strategies in different regions, and of considering malaria control programmes as part of a more general improvement in health infrastructure. They have also scaled back their optimism about eradication: the new international programme is called the Global Malaria *Action* (rather than 'Eradication') Plan (GMAP), and aims only for local elimination from particular countries. While GMAP does state that spending on malaria control can decrease as malaria is eliminated from some countries, so that money only needs to be spent making sure that it stays eliminated, current spending rates are about US$2.5 billion per year out of the US$8–10 billion that might be necessary for control and eradication—and this level of commitment will probably need to be maintained for decades.

Current efforts to control malaria have one new tool that was not available in the 1960s—insecticide-treated bed nets (ITNs) using pyrethroids, a class of insecticide that is safe for mammals (although toxic to fish). Pyrethroid-based ITNs were first deployed in the 1980s; long-lasting versions that can kill mosquitoes for five years beyond the six months' effectiveness of the original ITNs were deployed in the early 2000s. The idea of ITNs is not that different from indoor residual spraying—they kill mosquitoes that come indoors to bite humans—but they have the additional advantages of providing a physical as well as a chemical barrier, and working even in houses that have porous walls unsuitable for spraying. They have their logistical and cultural problems—for example, recipients have been known to use the nets for catching or drying fish rather than for malaria protection. However, given that no malaria control strategy is 100 per cent effective by itself, ITNs provide a vital addition to the malaria control arsenal.

One lesson of bed nets is that a long-lasting tool is nearly always better—more cost-effective and requiring less effort to deliver—than its short-lived counterpart. A bed net that needs to be replaced every five years is better, all other things equal, than a residual spraying programme that needs to be repeated every six months, even though the bed net only works when people sleep under it. A malaria vaccine, even if an imperfect and short-lived one, would be the compatibility filter analogue of bed nets; rather than treating people with artemisinin only after they got sick, you could just vaccinate them every few years. No malaria vaccine is yet (as of January 2015) available for use, but the currently most promising vaccine, which protected 25–50 per cent of children in clinical trials, is scheduled for use within the next few years. Researchers think it will be more cost-effective than bed nets in some areas.

We are still deeply ignorant about malarial parasites. Knowing more about the ancient history of different malaria strains—when, and from where, they entered the human population—would deepen our understanding of the zoonotic processes that give rise to new human strains. Knowing more about the current distribution and ecology of malaria in non-human primates could help us guess about the likelihood of future zoonotics. Increased sampling of wild populations, and faster and cheaper genomic scans of malaria and primate genomes, are helping to resolve the picture, but it is anyone's guess how completely we will ever understand either the ecology or the evolutionary history of malaria.

So what does the future hold for malaria control? There is some room for optimism. In the absence of major economic or political shocks to the developing world, or the emergence or re-emergence of pathogens that shift the focus away from malaria, the current efforts of many countries and foundations will continue to chip away at the burden of malaria over the next few decades. Elimination is possible in many areas, but malaria experts are at best cautiously optimistic about eradication.

Along with the evolution of mosquitoes and malaria, climate change and (more importantly) land use and economic change will continually move the target. No single magic bullet will solve the problem of malaria. Governments and agencies will have to deploy different combinations of the available tools (source control, residual spraying, bed nets, treatment, and eventually vaccine) in ways that are appropriate to the local situation.

Chapter 7
Batrachochytrium dendrobatidis

Batrachochytrium dendrobatidis (Bd), the subject of our last case study, differs in many ways from the earlier examples. This fungus is the first (and only) non-human pathogen we will discuss. Its genome is many times larger than the viruses and bacteria considered earlier, similar in size to the malaria protozoan's. It is a generalist pathogen, infecting hundreds of different amphibian species and driving some of them to extinction.

Most important, Bd is our first example of an *emerging* pathogen. In practice, the definition of an emerging pathogen is very broad; it essentially means a pathogen that we are newly concerned about for some reason. The pathogen may be truly novel, emerging through mutation. More commonly, zoonotic pathogens emerge when existing pathogens jump to a new species. We may also classify disease as emerging when we detect a previously known pathogen in a known host, but in a new geographic region. Alternatively, emergence might describe an increase in the virulence or transmission of an existing pathogen (due to mutation, or to some change in the host or the environment). Finally, hosts might have become less tolerant or less resistant due to a genetic or environmental change.

For emerging pathogens of humans, the prime suspect is zoonosis (as in HIV), sometimes combined with pathogen mutation (as in pandemic influenza). Human pathogens can also emerge when environmental change opens the environmental filter for an existing disease, as when mosquito vectors of dengue spread to North America, or when people increased their contact with Lyme-disease-bearing ticks by building houses in wooded areas.

Emerging diseases of non-human species are a concern for several reasons. Many non-human species are economically valuable; emerging disease can threaten our wallets or even our lives. Agricultural disease can threaten important crops. The Irish potato blight—a fungal pathogen that jumped from its origin in South America to Europe via North America—caused massive human mortality and fundamentally altered the history of Ireland.

Diseases can also affect economically important wild populations. The recent decline in honeybees, the causes of which are still hotly debated but are due in part to pathogen spread, has severely compromised the California almond crops they pollinate; chronic wasting disease in wild elk threatens to cost Canadian elk farmers millions of dollars. Hopefully, we would also care about the welfare of non-human organisms for selfless reasons—conserving non-human species is simply the right thing to do.

Bd in amphibians is definitely in the latter category—despite the economic value of some amphibian species in the frog-leg trade or in controlling pests, most of the species affected by Bd are economically unimportant. Nevertheless, we want to understand where Bd came from and discover how we can protect wild amphibian populations from its impact. The concepts and strategies we use in our efforts to determine Bd's origin can also serve as a case study for understanding and controlling future emerging diseases of non-human species.

Physiology and natural history

Bd is the black sheep of a large and otherwise mostly obscure family of fungi, the chytrids. While a few chytrid fungi attack other fungi or plants, most live harmlessly on decaying organic matter in aquatic environments. Bd is one of only two known chytrids that attacks vertebrates, the second being a salamander pathogen that was only discovered in 2013. (Chytrid biologists complain when people refer to Bd as '*the* chytrid fungus', feeling that this unfairly taints all chytrids with the misbehaviour of one species.) Bd lives on and within the skin of amphibians, especially on keratin, a hard protein found in the skin. Its life cycle alternates between structures called *thalli*—bottle-shaped cells that grow within the host's skin layers—and *zoospores*, small mobile cells that disperse from the thalli into the water, eventually landing either back on the same host's skin or on another host, thus spreading the infection.

We know very little about when and how Bd persists in the environment, away from its host organisms. This is a critical question if we want to understand how Bd spreads from one amphibian population to another; whether populations can recover or recolonize years after they have been locally extirpated by Bd; and how to design quarantine programmes to protect healthy populations from Bd. Given that many of Bd's relatives are free-living microbes, it would not be surprising if Bd also retained the capability to survive and grow in the environment. We know that Bd can persist in pure water for weeks or months, and thrives on the keratin found in amphibian skins, feathers, and the exoskeletons of insects and crustaceans such as shrimp and crayfish. At present, however, we don't know if Bd can persist for years, or move long distances, in the absence of a host.

Bd might persist between seasons on tadpoles. This life stage is more tolerant because tadpoles only have keratin around their mouths, which they may be able to discard in response to infection without dying. This form of *intraspecific reservoir*, where pathogens persist in a tolerant life stage of the same species, has also been suggested for other amphibian pathogens. Many kinds of tadpoles grow slower but don't die when infected with Bd; in other species tadpoles do die from Bd. The most important reservoirs and vectors of Bd infection are probably individuals from tolerant host species, which can harbour the fungi and pass them to new (or recovering) populations without being harmed themselves. Most amphibian communities contain tolerant hosts—researchers are still trying to understand what makes a host tolerant or intolerant of Bd. Some of the most important potential players are some species of crayfish, the American bullfrog, and the South African clawed frog *Xenopus laevis*. All of these species are widespread, have been able to invade new geographic regions with or without human help, and are tolerant of at least some strains of Bd.

Another item on the long list of things we don't know about Bd is how it kills its hosts. Researchers have speculated about various causes, including the production by Bd of some kind of toxin. However, most of the current evidence suggests that infected adult frogs typically die when the build up of Bd in their skin and its subsequent thickening and hardening prevents them from maintaining proper salt concentrations in their bodies, leading to death by cardiac arrest.

Amphibian species vary wildly in their susceptibility to Bd: wide variation in space, time, across species, and across communities is a hallmark of this emerging disease. Some of this variation may stem from differences in host defence. The immune systems of *Xenopus* frogs produce antibodies that recognize Bd, although there is only weak evidence at present that these proteins protect against the fungus. The evidence is stronger for the protective effect of the antimicrobial proteins that many species of frogs and toads secrete on to their skins; species whose

Batrochochytrium dendrobatidis

skin secretions inhibit Bd in a test tube also tend to survive infection better.

Finally, some species seem to have the capacity to generate behavioural 'fevers' in response to Bd, which grows fastest between seventeen and twenty-three degrees Celsius, but dies at temperatures of thirty degrees Celsius and higher. Although frogs are cold-blooded and can't shiver to raise their body temperatures, infected frogs can and do boost their body temperatures by spending more time in warm, sunny places, which appears to help them recover from Bd. Frogs can even be cured of Bd in the lab by putting them in warm environments for less than a day. Not all species can be cured in this way, suggesting that rather than harming Bd directly, warm temperatures may help frogs by improving their ability to produce antimicrobial proteins. Some of the variation among species could also be explained by the fact that different species are tested by different researchers, in different labs, using different experimental procedures.

Discovery

Ecologists discovered Bd in the late 1990s when frogs throughout eastern Australia and Central America started dying from mysterious causes. At about the same time, poison dart frogs in the US National Zoo also started dying. Veterinary researchers there got in touch with the few researchers in the world who knew anything about this previously obscure family of fungi. Between them they came up with a species description and a name based on the Latin name of poison dart frogs, *Dendrobates*: the genus name *Batrachochytrium* means 'chytrid that infects frogs and toads'.

One interesting sidelight of the discovery of Bd is the experience of Joyce Longcore, an expert on chytrid fungi. After keeping house and raising children for twenty years, Longcore went back to graduate school, receiving a PhD in mycology in 1991. As of 1997, just before the discovery of Bd, she looked set for a quiet career studying an obscure family of fungi. When Bd suddenly exploded in importance, she was the go-to person for information about the biology of chytrid fungi, and her career took off like a rocket. Since 1998 she has co-authored sixty-four papers with more than 3,700 total citations, making her a scientific star. Her story demonstrates the value of having the right knowledge at the right time. It also shows that seemingly arcane biological knowledge can suddenly become vital to understand a novel ecological situation.

Once it became clear that Bd was a previously unknown pathogen, biologists asked about its origins: had it arrived recently in the communities it was destroying, or had it lain dormant in those communities for millennia before suddenly beginning to cause harm? The ensuing debate between the *novel pathogen hypothesis* (NPH) and the *endemic pathogen hypothesis* (EPH), versions of which apply to most emerging diseases of wildlife, has been raging ever since. Although we have generated a huge amount of information about Bd and its interaction with amphibians in the two decades since its discovery, the debate continues: it seems that every time a new piece of research supports the NPH, another study follows quickly to add evidence for the EPH.

The NPH does not say that Bd is a new species—we know that it existed long before the 1990s. Rather, it says that Bd, or at least virulent strains of Bd, is new to the specific geographic areas in which we now see infected populations. If the NPH is true, then Bd must have moved into new areas around the time when disease-related die-offs were first observed. Under the NPH we would expect to see a clear spatial separation between regions where Bd has and has not yet arrived, rather than a patchwork of local regions with and without Bd-related die-offs. We should also be able to see a signature of its rapid spread in the spatial pattern of its genes, with high genetic diversity in regions where it has persisted for a long time and low genetic diversity in areas with recent disease outbreaks.

Batrachochytrium dendrobatidis

In contrast, the EPH asserts that the same strains of Bd have been present in amphibian communities, even the ones that have undergone recent disease outbreaks, for a long time. The *disease triangle*, an idea from plant epidemiology, says that a disease outbreak requires the presence of (1) a suitable host, (2) a pathogen, and (3) an environment in which the pathogen can overcome the encounter and compatibility filters in order to successfully spread from one host to another, and overcome tolerance to cause disease. The EPH says that the first two sides of the triangle have been in place for centuries or millennia, but that some change in the environment has recently opened the encounter and compatibility filters, or changed tolerance. Since Bd must (as far as we know now) be able to infect amphibian hosts in order to persist in the long term, it is not the encounter (transmission) or compatibility (resistance) filter that has opened; rather, proponents of the EPH think that changes in the environment have made hosts less tolerant of Bd, or equivalently have made Bd more virulent. To validate the EPH, we should not only fail to validate the predictions of the NPH (both the spatial distribution of Bd and its spatial pattern of genetic variation should be noisy and unpredictable); we should also be able to identify environmental covariates that predict whether hosts are tolerant/Bd is virulent in a particular community, and we should be able to find evidence that these covariates have changed recently in outbreak regions.

Before we go through the evidence for each hypothesis, it's worth keeping in mind that Bd emergence is complex—like all biological phenomena—and that the NPH and EPH are not mutually exclusive. It could be true both that Bd has recently moved into new geographic regions (as stated by the NPH), *and* that Bd has become more virulent or hosts have lost tolerance (as stated by the EPH).

We start with the historical and genetic evidence, which should help us determine when Bd arrived in different locations around the globe. As is the case with nearly all infectious diseases of wildlife, Bd existed long before biologists noticed it in amphibian communities. Unlike human diseases such as malaria or influenza, however, there are no historical records that can tell us where Bd was in the past—even if there had been ancient plagues where frogs and toads started dying in huge numbers, humans probably wouldn't have noticed. In fact, even when people *did* notice amphibian die-offs in the recent past, such as the disappearance of boreal toads from the mountains of Colorado in the 1970s, or the decline of *Atelopus* frogs in Central America in the late 1980s—declines that we attribute retrospectively to Bd—they attributed them to other causes, such as climate change or environmental stress coupled with bacterial outbreaks.

With the advent of good methods for identifying DNA—similar to those used in the archaeological discoveries of malaria in Egyptian mummies—researchers are able to go back in time by trying to detect Bd DNA on the skins of frogs borrowed from the collections of natural history museums. In both Colorado and Central America, they successfully recovered chytrid fungi from frog skins collected around the time of the outbreaks, making Bd-induced die-offs extremely plausible in hindsight. However, these results do not strongly support either the NPH or the EPH, since the researchers have not been able to show the *absence* of Bd in those areas in periods just before the outbreaks.

Researchers were excited to discover Bd DNA on the skins of *Xenopus* collected in South Africa in 1938. The early appearance of Bd associated with this widespread, tolerant species led them to propose the 'Out of Africa' hypothesis—the idea that the strains of Bd that would later originate the global Bd pandemic evolved in Africa some time prior to 1938 and only began to spread globally after a human pregnancy test based on *Xenopus* eggs was developed in the 1930s, leading to the export of thousands of *Xenopus* a year from South Africa. According to this hypothesis, the fungus would have had two decades to spread globally during

Batrachochytrium dendrobatidis

the 1940s and 1950s (before other pregnancy tests replaced the *Xenopus*-egg test), after which it gradually spread in new habitats, perhaps via other tolerant hosts.

However, these hypotheses are fragile—every time someone sets a new record by discovering Bd on an even older preserved amphibian skin, the story changes. Twin discoveries in 2013 and 2014 drastically shifted the grounds of the debate. First, researchers detected Bd on the skin of a bullfrog collected in 1928, in California. Bullfrogs had previously been suspected of spreading Bd across amphibian communities. This finding did not completely rule out the Out of Africa hypothesis, but it complicated it considerably. Since the Bd finding in California is too early for the pregnancy-test-driven export of *Xenopus* from Africa, either Bd would have to have jumped out of Africa more than ten years earlier via some other process, or the strain of Bd found in the Californian frog skin would have to represent a different (non-virulent) lineage. Next, in an even more sensational finding, a group of researchers discovered Bd on a quarter of the frogs from a huge collection from the Atlantic forest of Brazil going all the way back to 1894.

While researchers will keep pushing back these records, finding earlier and earlier occurrences of Bd around the globe, new discoveries get progressively harder as we go back in time simply because we have fewer museum specimens to test. Turning instead to the evidence from Bd's genome, we find again—as with so many aspects of Bd—that it's complicated. There are many families (lineages) of Bd, of which the most important (from our point of view) is the so-called *global pandemic lineage* (GPL), which contains all of the samples collected from amphibian populations that are in decline and a few others. In the first phylogenetic studies of Bd, GPL appeared to have the exact characteristics of a rapidly spreading pathogen family: the very low level of genetic variation among its members and lack of recognizable geographic pattern could both be explained by a process where pathogens colonized new communities much faster than they could evolve new genotypes characteristic of a particular region. More recent studies have once again complicated the picture. While the GPL still appears geographically chaotic, containing representative Bd strains from every region, a growing database and more thorough genome scans have shown researchers that it also contains considerable variation; the newest studies have increased the estimated age of the most recent ancestor of the GPL from as little as decades (consistent with an emerging pathogen that first arose around the time of *Xenopus* exports from Africa) to at least 10,000 years. Furthermore, the direct historical evidence from Brazilian frogs shows that, wherever the GPL originated, strains of Bd from that GPL lineage have been physically present in South America, apparently not leading to population declines and extinctions in amphibian communities, for a century.

We can hope that more analysis of museum skins, and still more thorough genome scans, may yet clarify the history of the lineages that are currently designated as the GPL. Deeper study may eventually succeed in dividing the GPL strains cleanly into one low-virulence group that has existed all over the world for millennia and a new, high-virulence group, possibly arising from hybridization between existing strains. As it spread from one geographic region to another over decades, this new group would have contributed to the retrospectively identified Bd-driven amphibian declines in Colorado in the 1970s, Central America in the 1980s, and eastern Australia and Central America in the 2000s.

On the other hand, the failure of the data to tell a compelling, uncomplicated story supporting the NPH may lead researchers back towards the EPH. In the early days—just after the discovery of the declines in Central America and Australia, and especially as it became obvious that the impact of Bd varied drastically from one community to another—researchers scrambled to find environmental changes that could explain the (apparently) sudden

Batrachochytrium dendrobatidis

virulence of Bd. One of the puzzling aspects of Bd-induced die-offs was that they often seemed to occur in high-elevation, pristine areas such as nature reserves—inconsistent with a story involving human-induced changes to the landscape. Two environmental factors that researchers initially thought might be interacting with Bd to cause die-offs, by stressing amphibians or depressing their immune responses, were pesticide contamination (possibly blown long distances from agricultural areas) and ultraviolet radiation (consistent with effects of elevation). Despite some associations with population declines, and some lab studies that have shown that ultraviolet radiation and pesticides can make Bd more virulent, these factors have not (yet) provided much power for predicting where and when Bd will strike amphibian communities.

Temperature has a stronger signal: it has been consistently associated with harmful effects of Bd both on individual animals in lab studies and on communities in nature. As already mentioned, studies have consistently shown that Bd does best within a narrow thermal window. Temperature can potentially explain the pattern of high-elevation die-offs, since temperatures are consistently cooler at higher elevations. However, while it may explain why lowland communities persist while their uphill neighbours are being destroyed by disease, it doesn't explain the temporal patterns—why have high-elevation communities only begun to be destroyed in the last few decades and not before, if (as often seems to be the case) Bd has been present for centuries? What has changed?

The most obvious candidate, and one that is always on environmentalists' radar, is human-induced climate change. Perhaps climate change, which we know severely affects ecological communities at high latitudes and high altitudes, has recently shifted conditions past a tipping point that allows Bd to spread and/or harm communities, either by increasing the growth rate of Bd (e.g. the zoospore production rate) or by lowering the compatibility filter of individual amphibians.

The climate change hypothesis has been controversial within the Bd research community. A high-profile 2006 study suggested that reduced daily temperature variation in the Central American highlands had facilitated outbreaks by allowing Bd to remain in its optimal thermal range more of the time. Other researchers claimed that this study made mistakes about important details such as the lag between temperature changes, Bd outbreaks, and community die-offs. Furthermore, the spatio-temporal pattern of the die-offs—which spread across Central America at a rate of hundreds of kilometres per year rather than affecting the entire region simultaneously—seemed more characteristic of the spread of a novel pathogen than of a change in regional climate. In support of the original hypothesis, subsequent analyses using the same climate and die-off data as well as additional climatic measurements suggested that changes in temperature variability, rather than mean temperature, were indeed associated with the die-offs, even after taking the spatial pattern of spread into account, and that die-offs might have been driven by local effects of the global decade-scale climate shift called El Niño, rather than by longer-term human-induced climate change. A global study of Bd die-offs found that annual precipitation is correlated with die-offs, although other similar studies failed to find a strong effect. While changes in climate may well contribute to the occurrence and impact of Bd outbreaks, they do not provide the smoking gun that the proponents of the EPH are looking for.

As the Bd story gets ever more complex, many biologists acknowledge that neither the NPH nor the EPH is ever going to tell the whole story. Are we any closer to understanding when, where, and why Bd occurs, and where it has dire consequences for amphibian populations? Yes. While science sometimes seems to go in a circle—researchers are still focused on the same hypotheses that framed the initial debates when Bd was first discovered—closer examination often shows, more encouragingly, that the path is more like an ever-narrowing helix. We return to the same arguments, but at a higher level, with a new level of

Batrachochytrium dendrobatidis

sophistication and drawing on new kinds of evidence. The extraction of Bd genomic data from recent and historical collections has given us a much deeper understanding of the distribution of Bd in space and time, and several new techniques promise more insights. Genomic data from amphibian hosts can provide evidence about past population bottlenecks; looking at the genes for antimicrobial proteins can suggest which species needed to defend themselves from Bd in the past. On the EPH side, proxies for past climate such as the isotopic composition of trees or soil (which reveal patterns of temperature and dryness) can give us a more complete picture of the way the host–pathogen–environment disease triangle worked in ancient environments.

Beyond intellectual satisfaction, does any of this information help us control Bd outbreaks or lessen their impact on amphibian communities? The NPH versus EPH debate has implications for Bd control strategies. If the NPH is correct, implying that the environment has *not* changed in important ways and that what's new is the presence of the pathogen, then conservationists should focus on preventing spread across communities. If the EPH is correct—i.e. the pathogen has been present all along but the environment has worsened—then we should worry about making the environment better for amphibians so that they can resist or tolerate Bd.

However, the dichotomy might be less practically useful than it first appears. *If* we can intervene to reverse the triggering change—the presence of the pathogen or the change in the environment—then we can protect amphibians. But it's not practical to remove Bd from the environment once it has arrived, and we can't change the occurrence of El Niño events or anthropogenic global change (at least not on a useful time scale). Conservation actions must be based on the overlap of actions that we think will attack the root causes of disease emergence, actions that are ethical (is it OK to cull some members of an endangered species to save the rest?), and actions that are logistically feasible.

Even without knowing anything about the disease, we can close the encounter filter by transporting individuals from the wild into disease-free, artificial habitats. The Amphibian Ark is a project that aims to preserve species by making sure that, no matter what happens in nature, we have some animals in captive breeding programmes that can (hopefully) be reintroduced into the wild once we have figured out how to control Bd. Biologists are already successfully rearing endangered species in captivity, but we don't know when or how we'll be able to reintroduce them. Captive rearing buys time, but eventually we either need to breed Bd-resistant variants of these species, or find a way to control Bd in nature. It also raises ethical issues: might we be harming endangered species by removing individuals from the wild? Could the existence of captive populations reduce the urgency we feel to deal with the problem? Is it OK to raise funds for conservation by raising additional captive animals for sale?

The next most direct way to try to save amphibians is by closing the compatibility filter for individuals in the wild. Antifungal drugs and temperature-raising treatments have worked to cure frogs of Bd in laboratory trials, and we may be able to scale these treatments up to capture, treat, and release enough individuals to save wild populations. Biologists have also proposed to treat amphibians with skin peptides from resistant species, or to treat individuals or even entire communities with a bacterium that produces antifungal compounds that suppress Bd. Very recently, researchers have discovered that exposing some amphibians to dead Bd in the lab can give them partial resistance to Bd, although it is too soon to know whether this finding can be used to develop a practical disease-fighting strategy.

The fight against Bd faces the same two fundamental problems as every other disease control and prevention programme—lack of knowledge and lack of resources. No matter how cute or interesting the victims are, diseases of wild animals will never command the same interest as human disease, so we will always

Batrachochytrium dendrobatidis

have fewer resources—and less knowledge, since resources are needed to acquire knowledge. We do have some advantages—we can cull animals if it looks like it will help us to control an outbreak, breed animals for disease tolerance or resistance, and induce experimental infections to evaluate treatments (all strategies that would be looked on unfavourably for human pathogen control). Since we haven't yet managed to deploy any disease control strategies in the field, we haven't yet had to worry about evolutionary countermeasures taken by the pathogen, although these are bound to happen once we start to take action.

Although infectious diseases of wild animals differ from those of humans in superficial ways, the physiological, ecological, and evolutionary dynamics that drive them are very similar. In the long run, analysing wildlife disease helps us understand the fundamental properties of infectious disease. It can help protect harvested or hunted populations that are economically valuable. Understanding how disease moves in natural populations may also provide early-warning systems to detect zoonotic diseases that can jump into humans. Perhaps most fundamentally, many biologists (including the authors of this book) feel that we have an ethical responsibility to preserve species when we can, especially when our actions may have contributed to the spread of diseases that threaten them.

Chapter 8
Looking ahead

This book has given a whirlwind tour of some important infectious diseases, their ecological and evolutionary principles, and how these principles inform treatment and control. We chose a few case studies we could fit into the book on the basis of socio-economic importance and ecological/evolutionary interest, covering a broad range of disease-causing taxa. Our choice was admittedly biased towards diseases we thought would be familiar to our readers.

We have regretfully omitted many infectious diseases that hurt many people, costing hundreds of thousands of lives, millions of disability-adjusted life years, and billions of dollars. Some examples include tuberculosis (the most important disease we have neglected), polio, and schistosomiasis (a parasitic disease that causes liver damage, mostly affecting people in sub-Saharan Africa). So many such diseases are rampant in less developed tropical countries that there is an entire category, 'neglected tropical diseases', and a scientific journal devoted to them.

We have also left out fascinating diseases that have shaped history. The bubonic plague, the greatest infectious killer ever, is now relatively easy to treat with antibiotics. Smallpox, the first disease to be eradicated in the wild by vaccination, destroyed native populations in the Americas and was used to facilitate European colonization. Finally, rinderpest, a cattle disease closely related to measles, may have transformed the landscape of east Africa by wiping out native wildlife and allowing the growth of shrubby vegetation which allowed tsetse flies, and through them a vector-borne disease called sleeping sickness or trypanosomiasis, to establish.

For the most part, we have focused on established diseases rather than emerging diseases, although HIV and Bd have emerged relatively recently, and the 2009 pandemic H1N1 strain of influenza could count as 'recently emerged'. We haven't had room to discuss emerging coronaviruses such as SARS or MERS; the henipaviruses such as Nipah virus that threaten to spill over from fruit bats in Australia and South East Asia; or emergent vector-borne diseases such as West Nile and dengue viruses, or the bacteria causing Lyme disease.

Finally, we have covered only a small range of the kinds of organisms that can cause infectious disease. Admittedly, viruses such as influenza and HIV, bacteria such as *Vibrio cholerae*, protozoans such as the malarial agent *Plasmodium falciparum*, and fungi such as *Batrachochytrium dendrobatidis* make up the vast majority of pathogenic agents. However, we have passed over multicellular parasites such as roundworms (nematodes) and flatworms (platyhelminths), which have traditionally been thought of separately from microparasitic infectious diseases (see Chapter 2), but which are driven by the same epidemiological, ecological, and evolutionary principles. Multicellular parasites and protozoans make up the majority of neglected tropical diseases. The general restriction of these diseases to relatively poor, less-developed countries, as well as their tendency to cause chronic debility rather than acute disease, contribute to their traditional relegation to a separate category.

In the past few decades, researchers have also discovered several absolutely new modes of infectious disease that seem almost like science fiction. The first, *prions* or transmissible infectious proteins, are misfolded proteins that can replicate within a host by catalysing the misfolding of other proteins to the prion form. Prion diseases such as scrapie, known to infect sheep since the 1700s, and chronic wasting disease, which was first detected infecting deer in Colorado in the 1960s, are probably transmitted from one animal to another when animals eat vegetation contaminated with prion proteins. Prion proteins get on to plants, completing the transmission cycle, through environmental contamination from animals' bodily fluids (saliva, faeces, or amniotic fluids) or when released into the soil from their cadavers.

Prion diseases hit the headlines in the 1990s with 'mad cow disease', officially called bovine spongiform encephalopathy (the condition is drily called 'variant Creutzfeldt–Jakob disease' when it occurs in humans). Along with the fear of contracting a disease that leads to fatal neurological degeneration, the British public was also fascinated by the grotesque cause of the outbreak, which was due to involuntary cannibalism among cattle. In order to promote their growth, the animals were fed protein supplements that included brain and spinal cord tissue from other cattle. Prion diseases can extremely rarely occur spontaneously in animals, or due to rare genetic defects; when the remains of these animals are mixed into the food of hundreds of other animals, catastrophe results. A similar but even more macabre epidemic of prion disease, involving human rather than bovine cannibalism, spread through the Fore people of Papua New Guinea starting in the early 20th century, in the wake of their adopting 'mortuary cannibalism'—the practice of ceremonially eating their dead relatives—and vanished again after the abandonment of cannibalism in the mid-20th century.

What is the outlook for the control of infectious diseases over the next few decades? What are the likely impacts of infectious disease on your health and welfare, or on your family's, from diseases that are already present, or from newly emerging ones? How will the ecology and evolution of disease change in the future?

The first thing we know is that 'plus ça change, plus c'est la même chose' (the more things change, the more they stay the same). Our understanding of how diseases are transmitted, and the development of vaccines and treatments that can close the compatibility filter, has revolutionized disease management, but the basic processes driving the disease ecosystem remain the same. Humans have had some resounding successes: we have completely eradicated smallpox and rinderpest, and we can realistically consider the possibility of polio and measles eradication even though the last steps are proving to be immensely difficult for social, political, and economic reasons. Even though it is hard to imagine eradicating HIV, we have developed treatments that allow infected people (at least those with access to good medical care) to tolerate the disease and live out their regular lifespan.

However, we have also lost ground. Tuberculosis has re-emerged, especially in conjunction with HIV; the first optimistic decades of malaria control ended in retreat; and new diseases such as Lyme disease, West Nile virus, and H1N1 influenza have continued to spill over from animal populations. Perhaps the scariest failures have been our glimpses of the potential of drug and antibiotic resistance in MRSA or malaria or multiply resistant tuberculosis, where we are once again forced to contemplate the spectre of untreatable diseases.

A future free of infectious disease is simply unrealistic. Living things have parasitized one another since the beginning of life itself, and no amount of intervention will alter that. New diseases will be created by mutation or recombination of existing ones and by spillover from animal populations, and existing diseases will continually evolve to escape our methods of control. What is attainable, however, is minimizing the impact of disease while understanding that it will always be with us. We *can* slow or stop pandemics, and we *can* reduce the amount of death and misery that diseases cause, even if we can never fully conquer them.

What has changed in our understanding of infectious diseases over the last fifty years? During that period, we moved from population-level treatment to individual treatment. What we have learned in this progression is that population-level treatment, in contrast to curing individuals after they have already been infected, is still invaluable in stopping disease. The simplest way to minimize the impact of disease is to minimize its incidence in the first place. We are learning that there is synergy between population-level and individual-level approaches to prevent disease. The phenomenon of herd immunity is one such example (see Chapter 2).

As our case studies have illustrated, the organisms that cause disease evolve. Tuberculosis is re-emerging in part because the bacteria that cause it have evolved antibiotic resistance. HIV evolved to survive better in humans following its host shift from other primates. But remember—mutations happen at random. So too do encounters between relatively harmless bacteria with bacteria or viruses carrying dangerous pathogenicity genes. Because of that inherent randomness, the fewer organisms that are present, the less likely it is that they will evolve to become more virulent. Think of it this way: if there are twenty viruses, and a mutation that makes them resistant to an antiviral agent happens only one in a million times, it's quite improbable that one of them will experience that rare mutation. But if there are a billion of them, the event is practically inevitable. So by keeping the numbers of organisms that infect us low through population-level interventions like effective vaccination or quarantine, we reduce the probability that they will evolve to become more dangerous. Again, an ounce of prevention is worth a pound of cure.

One of the lessons from past failures of disease control is that the miracles of modern molecular biology have limitations. Vaccines are simplest to develop when the human body already has a quick and effective immune response. For diseases like HIV, malaria, or tuberculosis that use evolutionary tricks such as costume-switching to evade the immune response, we may never be able to achieve the same cheap, effective vaccines that eradicated smallpox and have brought measles and polio to the brink of eradication.

Even as we have learned the limitations of magic bullets, we have new technological applications that can help with both detection of disease organisms and with healing. Identification of viruses or testing bacteria for antibiotic resistance used to take days or weeks. For example, virus classification involved careful microscopic inspection or time-consuming immunological techniques. Testing for resistance involved assessing the ability of bacteria to grow on plates containing various antibiotics. Now we can diagnose and characterize bacteria and viruses by sequencing their genomes within hours. Moreover, these techniques are no longer relegated to skilled technicians in laboratories; sequencing technologies suitable for unprocessed samples (such as saliva or blood) under field conditions are now available, and costs are dropping by the month. Such genotyping technologies may also be useful in bacterial infections, for tailoring the correct sort of phage to use against them as part of phage therapy.

Another lesson we have learned is the power, as well as the limitations, of changing human behaviour. We can easily close the encounter filter for many diseases by checking thoroughly for ticks after we go into the woods, stopping the exchange of bodily fluids with strangers, and staying home (or keeping our kids home) when we develop a cough. However, the practical and economic costs of changing our behaviour often mean that we keep exposing ourselves, and others, even when the solutions seem (on the surface) to be relatively simple and even when the consequences (such as contracting HIV) are dire. For you, the reader of this book, this is relatively good news; there are lots of simple ways that you can prevent your own infection, or, if you are infected, stop transmitting disease to others. But humans as a whole are stubborn creatures, and we have many conflicting priorities—earning a living or simply saving a little bit of time may often trump the practices that could save us, or others, from infection.

One of the important frontiers in disease control is figuring out better ways to honestly but effectively inform the public about the dangers of disease and the methods that are in their hands for controlling it. Sometimes the interests of the individual and the population diverge. For example, staying home from work when we're sick might be a bad individual decision on purely selfish grounds, because it costs us a day's pay or a boss's goodwill, even if it benefits our co-workers. We must do a better job at designing policies that encourage compliance with public health goals, using a sensible combination of carrots and sticks without unduly restricting individual freedoms.

The continuing pressure of humanity on the environment is another thing that has changed, but has also stayed the same. Urbanization and increased population growth increase the rates at which humans contract new pathogens, largely carried by animals. As we move into previously uncolonized habitats, or as we modify our environments, encounter rates with animals and the parasites they carry increase. This does not just apply to tropical diseases, but also to temperate diseases (recall Lyme disease). Humans are changing their environment in huge numbers of ways—cleaning our water, aggregating in modern mega-cities, clearing tropical forest—that will change our epidemiological landscapes both for better and for worse.

Epidemiologists are locked in an intense debate over the possible effects of the largest-scale uncontrolled experiment in history—the release of CO_2 from fossil fuels into the atmosphere, and the concomitant changes in global climate—on disease prevalence. On the one hand, there is no question that ecological change brings about epidemiological change; many species' ranges have already been observed to shift in response to climate change, and it makes sense that this would apply to insect vectors such as mosquitoes as well. In particular locations, such as the highlands of East Africa, increasing temperatures do indeed seem to have driven increases in the incidence of malaria. But the regional effects of climate change are complex, involving changes in variability, seasonal patterns and the hydrological cycle as well as the overall temperature. Add that to the complexity and unpredictability of interactions of ecological systems with regional climate, and other scientists say that although we can say with certainty that climate change will have *some* effect on disease, it is hard to know exactly what it will be.

Mosquitoes are an interesting problem. At first glance, getting rid of mosquitoes, at least the ones that we know vector particularly devastating diseases, seems like a good idea. Indeed, it has recently been argued that scientists have become too narrowly focused on problems of drug resistance of malaria, and that we could ignore that altogether if we decided to launch an attack on mosquitoes. Eliminating mosquitoes, however, requires interventions like draining wetlands and/or use of pesticides that devastate many other species. And, of course, mosquitoes become resistant to insecticides, even as malaria becomes resistant to antimalarial drugs. However, there's a larger point to be made here: we mustn't allow our thinking about infectious disease to stagnate. Overconfidence in any one solution (antimalarial drugs), or overfocus on any part of the multifaceted problem that is infectious disease (for example, solely on parasite resistance), limits our ability to solve any kind of problem.

Human health is not just about vanquishing wicked parasites, either with magic bullets, everyday practice, or even both. The parasites are embedded in the same natural system that we are. Though we have spent little time discussing it in this book, human sociology also has huge effects on the spread of infectious disease. In the New Testament, the Four Horsemen of the Apocalypse are War, Famine, Pestilence, and Death. There's a reason they are grouped together: perhaps the most effective way to rid ourselves of the worst of infectious disease would be to achieve world peace and global prosperity. Sadly, a broader understanding of ecology and evolution as they pertain to infectious disease seems rather more attainable.

Plus ça change, plus c'est la même chose. As we write, an outbreak of the Ebola virus has already killed thousands of people in western Africa. The emergence of Ebola underscores many of the points we have made throughout this book. Ebola is another example of a zoonotic disease. The virus likely came to us from bats, and while the shift from bats to people is uncommon, genetic analysis of a variety of strains tells us that it has happened several times. A technical fix to close the compatibility filter is not possible in the short term—as yet, we have no reliable vaccine or drug treatment for Ebola—but hydration and other support does seem to improve outcomes. Quarantines could be effective to close the encounter filter, but would have been most effective in the early stages of the epidemic. The local postcolonial infrastructure could not, and cannot, deal with the challenges of Ebola alone, and the attention of the world was elsewhere. This changed abruptly when, as with almost every other disease we have discussed, global travel enabled the spread of Ebola to North America and Europe. Thus far, transmission outside of Africa has been stopped promptly.

As with HIV, fear of Ebola has stigmatized the disease. People are understandably attempting to hide infection in themselves or their families, further complicating attempts to understand the scope and dynamics of the epidemic. There has been much discussion of the importance of not stigmatizing international healthcare workers returning to their homes following service in Africa, while dealing sensibly with the risk and fear of contagion among their compatriots. Fear has also led to food scarcity in the areas of sub-Saharan Africa where the epidemic is the worst, making quarantines even more challenging, and creating an additional crisis.

Ebola terrifies people in part because of the mode of transmission, and in part because the fatality rate, particularly in Africa, is high. All the bodily fluids of a person with an active Ebola infection—particularly anyone who has died from the disease—are loaded with infectious virus. However, Ebola's grisly mode of transmission means that the encounter filter is relatively small. You only need to come in contact with a few virus particles to get sick. But with the small encounter filter, people other than healthcare workers and those who take care of the dead are unlikely to become sick, because it is unlikely that they will come into contact with contaminated bodily fluids. (Unfortunately, traditional African customs often mean that many of a dead person's relatives come in contact with the body before and during the funeral.) For example, family members of Thomas Duncan, the first person to be diagnosed with Ebola in the US who subsequently died from the disease, did not become sick despite living with him for several days after he became contagious. Two of the nurses caring for Duncan in a hospital did become infected, but happily they recovered.

At the time of writing it is difficult to predict the trajectory of the Ebola epidemic. However, by the time this book is in the hands of a reader, it seems virtually inevitable that yet another infectious disease will be emerging. Plus ça change…Apologize politely to the masked stranger who comes to your party uninvited, and explain that s/he will have to indulge you in hand washing before visiting the buffet; regale your guests with True Stories of effective vaccination campaigns; and take any medications you are given as directed (but feel free to discuss them with your doctor!). We cannot hope to live in a world free of infectious disease, but if we act wisely, we can live more safely.

Further reading

Chapter 1: Introduction

Blake, John B. 1952. 'The Inoculation Controversy in Boston: 1721–1722'. *The New England Quarterly* 25 (4): 489–506.

Brault, Aaron C., Claire Y.-H. Huang, Stanley A. Langevin, Richard M. Kinney, Richard A. Bowen, Wanichaya N. Ramey, Nicholas A. Panella, Edward C. Holmes, Ann M. Powers, and Barry R. Miller. 2007. 'A Single Positively Selected West Nile Viral Mutation Confers Increased Virogenesis in American Crows'. *Nature Genetics* 39 (9): 1162–6.

Combes, Claude. 2005. *The Art of Being a Parasite*. Chicago, IL: University of Chicago Press.

Davies, Julian. 1995. 'Vicious Circles: Looking Back on Resistance Plasmids'. *Genetics* 139 (4): 1465.

D'Costa, Vanessa M., Christine E. King, Lindsay Kalan, Mariya Morar, Wilson W. L. Sung, Carsten Schwarz, Duane Froese, et al. 2011. 'Antibiotic Resistance Is Ancient'. *Nature* 477 (7365): 457–61.

Garrett, Laurie. 1995. *The Coming Plague: Newly Emerging Diseases in a World Out of Balance*. Reprint edition. New York: Penguin Books.

Mackowiak, Philip A., and Paul S. Sehdev. 2002. 'The Origin of Quarantine'. *Clinical Infectious Diseases* 35 (9): 1071–2.

Miranda, Mary Elizabeth G., and Noel Lee J. Miranda. 2011. 'Reston Ebolavirus in Humans and Animals in the Philippines: A Review'. *Journal of Infectious Diseases* 204 (suppl. 3): S757–60.

Stearns, Stephen C., and Jacob C. Koella. 2008. *Evolution in Health and Disease*. 2nd edition. Oxford; New York: Oxford University Press.

Chapter 2: Transmission at different scales

Bernoulli, Daniel, and Sally Blower. 2004. 'An Attempt at a New Analysis of the Mortality Caused by Smallpox and of the Advantages of Inoculation to Prevent It'. *Reviews in Medical Virology* 14 (5): 275–88.

Combes, Claude. 2004. *Parasitism: The Ecology and Evolution of Intimate Interactions.* Translated by Isaure de Buron and Vincent A. Connors. Chicago: University Of Chicago Press.

Hethcote, Herbert W. 1994. 'A Thousand and One Epidemic Models'. In *Frontiers in Mathematical Biology*, edited by Simon A. Levin, 504–15. Lecture Notes in Biomathematics 100. Berlin: Springer.

Keeling, Matthew James, and Pejman Rohani. 2008. *Modeling Infectious Diseases in Humans and Animals.* Princeton: Princeton University Press.

McGovern, B., E. Doyle, L. E. Fenelon, and S. F. FitzGerald. 2010. 'The Necktie As a Potential Vector of Infection: Are Doctors Happy to Do Without?' *The Journal of Hospital Infection* 75 (2): 138–9.

Thomas, Y., G. Vogel, W. Wunderli, P. Suter, M. Witschi, D. Koch, C. Tapparel, and L. Kaiser. 2008. 'Survival of Influenza Virus on Banknotes'. *Applied and Environmental Microbiology* 74 (10): 3002–7.

Chapter 3: Influenza

Adams, Patrick. 2012. 'The Influenza Enigma'. *Bulletin of the World Health Organization* 90 (4): 245.

Cohen, Jon, and David Malakoff. 2012. 'On Second Thought, Flu Papers Get Go-Ahead'. *Science* 336 (6077): 19–20.

Dushoff, Jonathan, Joshua B. Plotkin, Cécile Viboud, David J. D. Earn, and Lone Simonsen. 2006. 'Mortality Due to Influenza in the United States: An Annualized Regression Approach Using Multiple-Cause Mortality Data'. *American Journal of Epidemiology* 163 (2): 181–7.

Lipsitch, M., and C. Viboud. 2009. 'Influenza Seasonality: Lifting the Fog'. *Proceedings of the National Academy of Sciences* 106 (10): 3645–6.

Loeb, M., M.L. Russell, L. Moss, et al. 2010. 'Effect of Influenza Vaccination of Children on Infection Rates in Hutterite Communities: A Randomized Trial'. *JAMA* 303 (10): 943–50.

Mereckiene, Jolita, Suzanne Cotter, F. D'Ancona, C. Giambi, A. Nicoll, Daniel Levy-Bruhl, P. L. Lopalco, et al. 2010. 'Differences in National Influenza Vaccination Policies Across the European Union, Norway and Iceland 2008–2009'. <https://lenus.ie/hse/handle/10147/125883>.

Nobusawa, Eri, and Katsuhiko Sato. 2006. 'Comparison of the Mutation Rates of Human Influenza A and B Viruses'. *Journal of Virology* 80 (7): 3675–8.

Roach, Jared C., Gustavo Glusman, Arian F. A. Smit, Chad D. Huff, Robert Hubley, Paul T. Shannon, Lee Rowen, et al. 2010. 'Analysis of Genetic Inheritance in a Family Quartet by Whole-Genome Sequencing'. *Science* 328 (5978): 636–9.

Schuchat, Anne. 2010. 'CDC Response: H1N1 Presentation for Immunization Update 2010'. Centers for Disease Control and Prevention, 27 July. <http://www.cdc.gov/h1n1flu/imm_update_transcript.htm>.

Simonsen, Lone, Peter Spreeuwenberg, Roger Lustig, Robert J. Taylor, Douglas M. Fleming, Madelon Kroneman, Maria D. Van Kerkhove, Anthony W. Mounts, W. John Paget, and the GLaMOR Collaborating Teams. 2013. 'Global Mortality Estimates for the 2009 Influenza Pandemic from the GLaMOR Project: A Modeling Study'. *PLoS Med* 10 (11): e1001558.

Tamerius, James, Martha I. Nelson, Steven Z. Zhou, Cécile Viboud, Mark A. Miller, and Wladimir J. Alonso. 2011. 'Global Influenza Seasonality: Reconciling Patterns across Temperate and Tropical Regions'. *Environmental Health Perspectives* 119 (4): 439–45.

Chapter 4: HIV

Faria, Nuno R., Andrew Rambaut, Marc A. Suchard, Guy Baele, Trevor Bedford, Melissa J. Ward, Andrew J. Tatem, et al. 2014. 'The Early Spread and Epidemic Ignition of HIV-1 in Human Populations'. *Science* 346 (6205): 56–61.

Frank, Steven A. 2002. *Immunology and Evolution of Infectious Disease*. Princeton, NJ: Princeton University Press.

Fraser, C., K. Lythgoe, G. E. Leventhal, G. Shirreff, T. D. Hollingsworth, S. Alizon, and S. Bonhoeffer. 2014. 'Virulence and Pathogenesis of HIV-1 Infection: An Evolutionary Perspective'. *Science* 343 (6177).

Holmes, Edward C. 2009. *The Evolution and Emergence of RNA Viruses*. Oxford: Oxford University Press.

Marx, Preston A., Phillip G. Alcabes, and Ernest Drucker. 2001. 'Serial Human Passage of Simian Immunodeficiency Virus by Unsterile Injections and the Emergence of Epidemic Human Immunodeficiency Virus in Africa'. *Philosophical Transactions of the Royal Society B: Biological Sciences* 356 (1410): 911–20.

Mild, Mattias, Rebecca R. Gray, Anders Kvist, Philippe Lemey, Maureen M. Goodenow, Eva Maria Fenyö, Jan Albert, Marco Salemi, Joakim Esbjörnsson, and Patrik Medstrand. 2013. 'High Intrapatient HIV-1 Evolutionary Rate Is Associated with CCR5-to-CXCR4 Coreceptor Switch'. *Infection, Genetics and Evolution* 19 (October): 369–77.

Müller, Viktor, and Sebastian Bonhoeffer. 2008. 'Intra-Host Dynamics and Evolution of HIV Infection'. In *Origin and Evolution of Viruses*, 2nd edition, edited by Esteban Domingo, Colin R. Parrish, and John J. Holland, 279–301. London: Academic Press.

Novembre, John, and Eunjung Han. 2012. 'Human Population Structure and the Adaptive Response to Pathogen-Induced Selection Pressures'. *Philosophical Transactions of the Royal Society B: Biological Sciences* 367 (1590): 878–86.

Sharp, Paul M., and Beatrice H. Hahn. 2011. 'Origins of HIV and the AIDS Pandemic'. *Cold Spring Harbor Perspectives in Medicine* 1 (1): a006841.

Chapter 5: Cholera

Colwell, Rita R. 1996. 'Global Climate and Infectious Disease: The Cholera Paradigm'. *Science*, New Series, 274 (5295): 2025–31.

Jubair, Mohamma, J. Glenn Morris, and Afsar Ali. 2012. 'Survival of *Vibrio cholerae* in Nutrient-Poor Environments Is Associated with a Novel "Persister" Phenotype'. *PLoS ONE* 7 (9): e45187.

Kaper, J. B., J. G. Morris, and M. M. Levine. 1995. 'Cholera'. *Clinical Microbiology Reviews* 8 (1): 48–86.

Kitaoka, Maya, Sarah T. Miyata, Daniel Unterweger, and Stefan Pukatzki. 2011. 'Antibiotic Resistance Mechanisms of *Vibrio cholerae*'. *Journal of Medical Microbiology* 60 (4): 397–407.

Morris, J. Glenn. 2011. 'Cholera: Modern Pandemic Disease of Ancient Lineage'. *Emerging Infectious Diseases* 17 (11).

Nelson, Eric J., Ashrafuzzaman Chowdhury, James Flynn, Stefan Schild, Lori Bourassa, Yue Shao, Regina C. LaRocque, Stephen B. Calderwood, Firdausi Qadri, and Andrew Camilli. 2008.

'Transmission of *Vibrio cholerae* Is Antagonized by Lytic Phage and Entry into the Aquatic Environment'. *PLoS Pathog* 4 (10): e1000187.

Zuger, Abigail. 2011. 'Small Fixes: Folding Saris to Filter Cholera-Contaminated Water'. *The New York Times*, 26 September. <http://www.nytimes.com/2011/09/27/health/27sari.html>.

Chapter 6: Malaria

Faust, E. C. 1951. 'The History of Malaria in the United States'. *American Scientist* 39 (1): 121–30.

Gladwell, Malcolm. 2001. 'The Mosquito Killer'. *The New Yorker*, 2 July. <http://www.newyorker.com/magazine/2001/07/02/the-mosquito-killer>.

Hedrick, Philip W. 2012. 'Resistance to Malaria in Humans: The Impact of Strong, Recent Selection'. *Malaria Journal* 11 (October): 349.

Kantele, Anu, and T. Sakari Jokiranta. 2011. 'Review of Cases with the Emerging Fifth Human Malaria Parasite, *Plasmodium knowlesi*'. *Clinical Infectious Diseases* 52 (11): 1356–62.

Klayman, D. L. 1985. 'Qinghaosu (artemisinin): An Antimalarial Drug from China'. *Science* 228 (4703): 1049–55.

Krief, Sabrina, Ananias A. Escalante, M. Andreina Pacheco, Lawrence Mugisha, Claudine André, Michel Halbwax, Anne Fischer, et al. 2010. 'On the Diversity of Malaria Parasites in African Apes and the Origin of *Plasmodium falciparum* from Bonobos'. *PLoS Pathog* 6 (2): e1000765.

Lalremruata, Albert, Markus Ball, Raffaella Bianucci, Beatrix Welte, Andreas G. Nerlich, Jürgen F. J. Kun, and Carsten M. Pusch. 2013. 'Molecular Identification of Falciparum Malaria and Human Tuberculosis Co-Infections in Mummies from the Fayum Depression (Lower Egypt)'. *PLoS ONE* 8 (4): e60307.

Liu, Weimin, Yingying Li, Gerald H. Learn, Rebecca S. Rudicell, Joel D. Robertson, Brandon F. Keele, Jean-Bosco N. Ndjango, et al. 2010a. 'Origin of the Human Malaria Parasite *Plasmodium falciparum* in Gorillas'. *Nature* 467 (7314): 420–5.

Liu, Weimin, Yingying Li, Katharina S. Shaw, Gerald H. Learn, Lindsey J. Plenderleith, Jordan A. Malenke, Sesh A. Sundararaman, et al. 2014. 'African Origin of the Malaria Parasite *Plasmodium vivax*'. *Nature Communications* 5 (February).

Nosten, François H. 2014. 'How to Beat Malaria, Once and for All'. *The New York Times*, 7 June. <http://www.nytimes.com/2014/06/08/opinion/sunday/how-to-beat-malaria-once-and-for-all.html>.

Outlaw, Diana C., and Robert E. Ricklefs. 2011. 'Rerooting the Evolutionary Tree of Malaria Parasites'. *Proceedings of the National Academy of Sciences* 108 (32): 13183–7.

Piel, Frédéric B., Anand P. Patil, Rosalind E. Howes, Oscar A. Nyangiri, Peter W. Gething, Thomas N. Williams, David J. Weatherall, and Simon I. Hay. 2010. 'Global Distribution of the Sickle Cell Gene and Geographical Confirmation of the Malaria Hypothesis'. *Nature Communications* 1: 104.

Poinar, G., and S. R. Telford. 2005. '*Paleohaemoproteus burmacis* Gen. N., Sp. N. (Haemospororida: Plasmodiidae) from an Early Cretaceous Biting Midge (Diptera: Ceratopogonidae)'. *Parasitology* 131 (01): 79–84.

Rich, Stephen M., Monica C. Licht, Richard R. Hudson, and Francisco J. Ayala. 1998. 'Malaria's Eve: Evidence of a Recent Population Bottleneck throughout the World Populations of *Plasmodium falciparum*'. *Proceedings of the National Academy of Sciences* 95 (8): 4425–30.

Rich, Stephen M., and Guang Xu. 2011. 'Resolving the Phylogeny of Malaria Parasites'. *Proceedings of the National Academy of Sciences* 108 (32): 12973–4.

Tishkoff, Sarah A., Robert Varkonyi, Nelie Cahinhinan, Salem Abbes, George Argyropoulos, Giovanni Destro-Bisol, Anthi Drousiotou, et al. 2001. 'Haplotype Diversity and Linkage Disequilibrium at Human G6PD: Recent Origin of Alleles that Confer Malarial Resistance'. *Science* 293 (5529): 455–62.

Webb, James L. A. 2009. 'The Long Shadow of Malaria Interventions in Tropical Africa'. *The Lancet* 374 (9705): 1883–4.

Chapter 7: *Batrachochytrium dendrobatidis*

Blaustein, Andrew R., John M. Romansic, Erin A. Scheessele, Barbara A. Han, Allan P. Pessier, and Joyce E. Longcore. 2005. 'Interspecific Variation in Susceptibility of Frog Tadpoles to the Pathogenic Fungus *Batrachochytrium dendrobatidis*. *Conservation Biology* 19 (5): 1460–8.

Briggs, Cheryl J., Vance T. Vredenburg, Roland A. Knapp, and Lara J. Rachowicz. 2005. 'Investigating the Population-Level Effects of

Chytridiomycosis: An Emerging Infectious Disease of Amphibians'. *Ecology* 86 (12): 3149–59.

Burke, Katie L. 2013. 'Probiotics for Frogs'. *American Scientist* 100 (3): 190.

Fisher, Matthew C., Trenton W. J. Garner, and Susan F. Walker. 2009. 'Global Emergence of *Batrachochytrium dendrobatidis* and Amphibian Chytridiomycosis in Space, Time, and Host'. *Annual Review of Microbiology* 63 (1): 291–310.

Gervasi, Stephanie S., Jenny Urbina, Jessica Hua, Tara Chestnut, Rick A. Relyea, and Andrew R. Blaustein. 2013. 'Experimental Evidence for American Bullfrog (*Lithobates catesbeianus*) Susceptibility to Chytrid Fungus (*Batrachochytrium dendrobatidis*)'. *EcoHealth* 10 (2): 166–71.

Kilpatrick, A. Marm, Cheryl J. Briggs, and Peter Daszak. 2010. 'The Ecology and Impact of Chytridiomycosis: An Emerging Disease of Amphibians'. *Trends in Ecology & Evolution* 25 (2): 109–18.

Lips, Karen R., Jay Diffendorfer, Joseph R. Mendelson III, and Michael W. Sears. 2008. 'Riding the Wave: Reconciling the Roles of Disease and Climate Change in Amphibian Declines'. *PLoS Biol* 6 (3): e72.

Martel, An, Annemarieke Spitzen-van der Sluijs, Mark Blooi, Wim Bert, Richard Ducatelle, Matthew C. Fisher, Antonius Woeltjes, et al. 2013. '*Batrachochytrium salamandrivorans* Sp. Nov. Causes Lethal Chytridiomycosis in Amphibians'. *Proceedings of the National Academy of Sciences* 110 (38): 15325–9.

McMahon, Taegan A., Laura A. Brannelly, Matthew W. H. Chatfield, Pieter T. J. Johnson, Maxwell B. Joseph, Valerie J. McKenzie, Corinne L. Richards-Zawacki, Matthew D. Venesky, and Jason R. Rohr. 2013. 'Chytrid Fungus *Batrachochytrium dendrobatidis* Has Nonamphibian Hosts and Releases Chemicals that Cause Pathology in the Absence of Infection'. *Proceedings of the National Academy of Sciences* 110 (1): 210–15.

McMahon, Taegan A., Brittany F. Sears, Matthew D. Venesky, Scott M. Bessler, Jenise M. Brown, Kaitlin Deutsch, Neal T. Halstead, et al. 2014. 'Amphibians Acquire Resistance to Live and Dead Fungus Overcoming Fungal Immunosuppression'. *Nature* 511 (7508): 224–7.

Rachowicz, Lara J., Roland A. Knapp, Jess A. T. Morgan, Mary J. Stice, Vance T. Vredenburg, John M. Parker, and Cheryl J. Briggs. 2006. 'Emerging Infectious Disease As a Proximate Cause of Amphibian Mass Mortality'. *Ecology* 87 (7): 1671–83.

Rodriguez, D., C. G. Becker, N. C. Pupin, C. F. B. Haddad, and K. R. Zamudio. 2014. 'Long-Term Endemism of Two Highly Divergent Lineages of the Amphibian-Killing Fungus in the Atlantic Forest of Brazil'. *Molecular Ecology* 23 (4): 774–87.

Rosenblum, Erica Bree, Timothy Y. James, Kelly R. Zamudio, Thomas J. Poorten, Dan Ilut, David Rodriguez, Jonathan M. Eastman, et al. 2013. 'Complex History of the Amphibian-Killing Chytrid Fungus Revealed with Genome Resequencing Data'. *Proceedings of the National Academy of Sciences* 110 (23): 9385–90.

Rohr, Jason R., and Thomas R. Raffel. 2010. 'Linking Global Climate and Temperature Variability to Widespread Amphibian Declines Putatively Caused by Disease'. *Proceedings of the National Academy of Sciences* 107 (18): 8269–74.

Chapter 8: Looking ahead

Brown, P., R. G. Will, R. Bradley, D. M. Asher, and L. Detwiler. 2001. 'Bovine Spongiform Encephalopathy and Variant Creutzfeldt-Jakob Disease: Background, Evolution, and Current Concerns'. *Emerging Infectious Diseases* 7 (1): 6–16.

Fisman, David, Edwin Khoo, and Ashleigh Tuite. 2014. 'Early Epidemic Dynamics of the West African 2014 Ebola Outbreak: Estimates Derived with a Simple Two-Parameter Model'. *PLOS Currents Outbreaks*. 8 September. Edition 1.

Hewlett, Barry, and Bonnie Hewlett. 2007. *Ebola, Culture and Politics: The Anthropology of an Emerging Disease*. Andover: Cengage Learning.

Reiter, Paul, Christopher J. Thomas, Peter M. Atkinson, Simon I. Hay, Sarah E. Randolph, David J. Rogers, G. Dennis Shanks, Robert W. Snow, and Andrew Spielman. 2004. 'Global Warming and Malaria: A Call for Accuracy'. *The Lancet Infectious Diseases* 4 (6): 323–4.

Suzuki, Y., and T. Gojobori. 1997. 'The Origin and Evolution of Ebola and Marburg Viruses'. *Molecular Biology and Evolution* 14 (8): 800–6.

Index

SOCIAL MEDIA
Very Short Introduction

Join our community
www.oup.com/vsi

- Join us online at the official Very Short Introductions **Facebook** page.
- Access the thoughts and musings of our authors with our online **blog**.
- Sign up for our monthly **e-newsletter** to receive information on all new titles publishing that month.
- Browse the full range of Very Short Introductions online.
- Read **extracts** from the Introductions for free.
- Visit our library of **Reading Guides**. These guides, written by our expert authors will help you to question again, why you think what you think.
- If you are a teacher or lecturer you can order inspection copies quickly and simply via our website.

ONLINE CATALOGUE
A Very Short Introduction

Our online catalogue is designed to make it easy to find your ideal Very Short Introduction. View the entire collection by subject area, watch author videos, read sample chapters, and download reading guides.

http://fds.oup.com/www.oup.co.uk/general/vsi/index.html

HIV/AIDS
A Very Short Introduction
Alan Whiteside

HIV/AIDS is without doubt the worst epidemic to hit humankind since the Black Death. The first case was identified in 1981; by 2004 it was estimated that about 40 million people were living with the disease, and about 20 million had died. The news is not all bleak though. There have been unprecedented breakthroughs in understanding diseases and developing drugs. Because the disease is so closely linked to sexual activity and drug use, the need to understand and change behaviour has caused us to reassess what it means to be human and how we should operate in the globalising world. This *Very Short Introduction* provides an introduction to the disease, tackling the science, the international and local politics, the fascinating demographics, and the devastating consequences of the disease, and explores how we have—and must—respond.

'It won't make you an expert. But you'll know what you're talking about and you'll have a better idea of all the work we still have to do to wrestle this monster to the ground.'

Aids-free world website.